The Human Nociceptive Withdrawal Reflex

The Human Nociceptive Withdrawal Reflex

Improved Understanding and Optimization of Reflex Elicitation and Recording

PhD Thesis by

Ken Steffen Frahm

*Center for Sensory-Motor Interaction,
Department of Health Science and Technology,
Aalborg University, Denmark*

River Publishers

Aalborg

ISBN 978-87-92982-69-8 (paperback)
ISBN 978-87-92982-68-1 (e-book)

Published, sold and distributed by:
River Publishers
Niels Jernes Vej 10
9220 Aalborg Ø
Denmark

Tel.: +45369953197
www.riverpublishers.com

Contents

Preface

The work presented in this PhD thesis is the result of research carried out at the Center for Sensory-Motor interaction (SMI) at Aalborg University (Denmark) in the period from September 2009 to March 2013. The research was supported by the Danish Research Council for Technology and Production (FTP). During this project five months, between April and August 2011, were spent at Duke University, Durham, NC, USA in collaboration with Dr. Warren M. Grill.

This thesis investigates the basic methodology behind the human nociceptive withdrawal reflex (NWR). The aims of this thesis were to investigate this methodology as a potential way of reducing the variability of NWR assessment and, if possible try, to discover methods which could help to reduce this variability. In order to fulfill these aims electrophysiological experiments, advanced mathematical modeling and anatomical studies were applied to investigate the elicitation and recording of the NWR.

This thesis contains four chapters. The Introduction presents the reader to the background and motivation for this project and gives a general overview of the PhD thesis. The Methods chapter introduces the used methods and elaborates the background for choosing them. The Results chapter presents and discusses the main findings in this thesis; in addition, all these findings are further elaborated in the original papers. The Conclusions chapter sums up the main findings and the impact on the state of the art, and finally looks at the perspectives towards future studies.

The thesis is based on three original papers that all are either published in, or submitted to, peer-reviewed journals. In addition one submitted peer-reviewed paper and several conference abstracts were based on the research conducted in this project.

Acknowledgements

During my time as a PhD student, I have enjoyed the support of so many people, all of whom I can never thank enough. First of all I would like to express my deepest gratitude towards my supervisor Professor, Dr.Scient., Ole K. Andersen for invaluable discussions and fantastic guidance throughout my PhD. His insight, support and inspiration and at some times immense patience has meant so much to me during this project. I could never have imagined a better supervisor for my PhD.

Secondly I wish to thank all of my co-authors and collaborators. Especially Associate Professor Carsten Dahl Mørch for his help and comments through the majority of this project. We have shared many good discussions and developed ideas for this thesis for this I am truly grateful. Furthermore, I wish to thank Professor Dario Farina and fellow PhD student Michael B. Jensen for their collaboration and fruitful discussions during the design, conducting and analysis of the EMG experiments. I wish to thank Professor Warren M. Grill for making my stay at Duke University possible and welcoming me in his lab. In addition, I wish to thank Postdoctoral fellow George C. McConnell and Assistant Research Professor Paul B. Yoo for their help during the nerve staining studies at Duke University. I am deeply grateful to Associate Professor Kristian Hennings for his help and valuable comments, and especially his insight during the nerve modeling.

I also want to express my appreciation to Associate Professor John Hansen and Knud Larsen who both have been a fantastic help for me with their Labview support and technical insight.

My deepest gratitude goes to all my dear friends and valued colleagues at SMI and HST, both previous and present, in particular Assistant Professor José Biurrun Manresa for his help throughout this project. I also wish to thank all the technical and administrative staff for their kind being and professional support, especially Susanne Nielsen Lundis for her help with this thesis.

And off course my most treasured colleague of all, Saba, who have been a tremendous support during this period and have shown extraordinarily patience with me. Without her continuous love, support and never-failing encouragements this thesis would not have been. I cannot describe her importance during my time as a PhD student both professionally and personally.

Finally, I wish to thank my entire family especially my parents and my sisters for their understanding, love and support during the past years. Furthermore, a special thanks to my sister Henriette for proof reading this thesis and continuous consulting and support during my life as a PhD student.

From the bottom of my heart thanks to all mentioned and also to all of you who slipped my lacking memory

Steffen

Aalborg 2013

English summary

The human nociceptive withdrawal reflex (NWR) has been the subject of substantial research which has shown that this reflex is a valuable tool in pain research as the reflex is highly correlated with the subjective pain perception. Furthermore, studies have also shown that the reflex can help to quantify to what degree a patient may suffer from central sensitization associated with many chronic pain conditions. Today, there exist no objective methods for probing spinal sensitization and thus the NWR could provide a valuable diagnostic tool and for assessment of treatment efficacy in patients suffering from chronic pain. However, the intra and inter-subject variability of the RRF method is still too high to be routinely used in clinic. The aim of this PhD was to investigate and if possible optimize the basic methodology for assessment of the NWR, which includes both the recording method (study I) and the techniques for eliciting the NWR (study II and III).

The three studies found ways of reducing crosstalk when recording the NWR using EMG (study I) based on double differential recordings (DD). In addition several parameters were examined to give a recommendation for the more optimal NWR recording strategy, e.g. an inter-electrode distance (IED) of 15-20 mm seems to be the optimal value. EMG recordings with IEDs of 15-20 mm detected 92-96 % of all reflexes in the DD recordings from the tibialis anterior muscle (TA) and 64-72 % of all reflexes in the DD recordings from the soleus muscle (SOL). Furthermore, an IED of 15-20 mm resulted in less than 2 % false detections of TA reflexes detected as SOL reflexes and less than 5 % false detections of SOL reflexes detected as TA reflexes. Study II documented that stimulation across the sole of the foot appeared to result in different levels of neural activation (significantly lower use of the McGill descriptor Sharp at the heel, indicating a lower degree of Aδ fiber activation). The thicker skin at the heel and pads caused large differences in the volume conductor, which could be seen as an impedance difference of more than 75 % between the heel and arch. These differences in the volume conductor resulted in an activation-function up to 231 % higher in the arch than in the heel. However, more advanced neural modeling, including realistic representation of the nerve morphology, indicated that volume conductor differences was not sufficient to explain the differences (study III). Moreover, there was significantly higher innervation density in dorsum of the foot than in the sole of the foot. But no evidence was found for different innervation density across the sole of the foot itself (study III). These findings suggest that the investigated peripheral mechanisms like skin thickness and nerve innervation density cannot alone explain the varying neural activation across the sole of the foot for equal stimulus intensities. This may suggest a possible central component modulating the afferent input, but this needs further investigation.

Future research on the NWR should focus on whether the optimal recording setup suggested by the present studies in fact reduces the NWR variability and thereby also improves the validity of the NWR method for probing central sensitization. Furthermore, since study II and III did not recommend specific parameters for improving the stimulation setup for eliciting the NWR future research is also needed in this area.

Danish summary / Dansk opsummering

Den humane nociceptive afværgerefleks (NWR) har været genstand for omfattende forskning, hvilket har vist at NWR er et vigtigt værktøj i smerteforskning, da refleksen i høj grad er korreleret til den subjektive smerteopfattelse. Ydermere har studier vist, at NWR kan hjælpe med kvantificere, i hvor høj grad en patient lider af central sensibilisering. Sådanne sensibiliseringer er associeret med mange typer kroniske smerter. I dag findes der ingen objektiv metode til at undersøge den spinale nociception og derfor er det muligt, at NWR kan bruges som et værdifuldt diagnostisk værktøj samt til at vurdere behandlingseffektiviteten i patienter med kroniske smerter. Dog lider NWR metoden af høj intra- og inter-patient variabilitet, hvilket hidtil har gjort den uegnet til daglig klinisk brug. Formålet med denne ph.d. var at undersøge, hvorvidt det er muligt at optimere den grundlæggende metode for NWR måling (studie I) og udløsning af NWR via elektrisk stimulation (studie II og III).

De tre studier fandt metoder til at reducere crosstalk under NWR optagelse vha. dobbelt differentierede EMG optagelser (DD) (studie I). Derudover blev adskillige parametre undersøgt for at opnå en mere optimal optageteknik. Bl.a. blev inter-elektrode-afstanden (IED) undersøgt og en IED på 15-20 mm fremstod som det optimale valg. EMG optagelser ved en IED på 15-20 mm gav en detektionsrate på 92-96% ved DD optagelse af reflekser fra m. tibilias anterior (TA) og en detektionsrate på 64-72 % ved DD optagelse af reflekser fra m. soleus (SOL). Ydermere resulterede en IED på 15-20 mm i mindre end 2 % fejldetektioner af TA reflekser detekteret som SOL reflekser og mindre end 5 % fejldetektioner af SOL reflekser detekteret som TA reflekser. Studie II dokumenterede, at stimulation i forskellige steder på fodsålen tilsyneladende resulterede i forskellige niveauer af neural aktivering (signikant lavere scoring af McGill-værdien Sharp, hvilket indikerer en lavere grad af Aδ fiber aktivering). Den tykkere hud på hæl og trædepuder gav anledning til store forskelle i en volumenledermodel, hvilket resulterede i impedansforskel på mere end 75 % imellem hælen og svangen. Disse forskelle i volumenledning resulterede i en aktiveringsfunktion, der var op til 231 % højere i svangen end på hælen. Dog viste mere avanceret nervemodellering som inkluderede realistisk nervemorfologi, at forskelle i hudtykkelse og deraf ændret volumenledning ikke kunne forklare variationen i nerveaktivering ved ens stimulationsstyrke (studie III). Derudover blev der fundet signifikante forskelle i nerveinnerveringsdensitet imellem fodsålen og fodryggen. Men der blev ikke fundet signifikante forskelle i nerveinnerveringsdensitet indenfor selve fodsålen (studie III). Disse fund indikerer, at de undersøgte perifere mekanismer ikke alene kan forklare de forskelle i nerveaktivering ved elektrisk stimulation over fodsålen. Derfor er det tænkeligt, at en central mekanisme modulerer det afferente input, hvilket dog kræver yderligere forskning.

Fremtidig forskning indenfor NWR bør fokusere på, hvorvidt den optageteknik forslået i denne afhandling kan reducere NWR variabilitet og dermed forbedre validiteten af NWR metoden til at undersøge central sensibilisering. Da studie II og III ikke direkte kom til en anbefaling af ændrede parametre til at opnå bedre NWR fremkaldelse, er fremtidig forskning indenfor dette felt nødvendigt.

List of abbreviations

AF	activation function
ANOVA	analysis of variance
AP	action potential
DD	double differential
EEG	electroencephalography
EMG	electromyography
FEM	finite element method
GM	gastrocnemius
IED	inter electrode distance
iEMG	intramuscular electromyography
MPQ	McGill pain questionnaire
Na_v	voltage gated sodium channel
NWR	nociceptive withdrawal reflex
per-thr	perception threshold
RM ANOVA	repeated measures analysis of variance
RMS	root mean square
RRF	reflex receptive field
SC	stratum corneum
sEMG	surface electromyography
SD	single differential
SF-MPQ	short form McGill pain questionnaire
SOL	soleus
TA	tibialis anterior
VAS	visual analog scale

Introduction

Chronic pain is a major health concern in today's world. The prevalence in developed countries is very high; usually between 17 and 20 % of the population (Blyth et al. 2001; Eriksen & Sjogren 2006), this means that a large proportion of the population will suffer from chronic pain at some point in their life. In many cases the pain conditions are very costly and invalidating; both for the individual, but also for the society, as the socio-economical effects are enormous. The incidence rate in Denmark was found to be 1.8 % per year in the period from 1994 to 2000 (Eriksen & Sjogren 2006), and it is expected that in Denmark alone there are 5-7000 new individuals suffering from chronic pain each year (Eriksen & Sjogren 2006).

In many pain patients the cause of the pain remains unknown to the clinicians. Therefore, the treatment for many pain patients is simply of a palliative nature (Eriksen & Sjogren 2006). This treatment usually requires the use of drugs like opioids and similar analgesics which might relieve the symptoms, but not the causes for the chronic pain. In addition, the use of such drugs is associated with a number of disadvantages, e.g. the risk of abuse and addiction.

Often the chronic pain is associated with a pathological hypersensitivity in the spinal cord and the rest of the central nervous system (CNS), so-called central sensitization (Woolf 1983). Central sensitization is defined as increased nociceptive neuronal excitability in the CNS for both normal and subthreshold stimuli (Loeser & Treede 2008). Woolf discovered that tissue damage will not only affect the excitability of the neurons from the ipsilateral side but also the contralateral neurons will have increased excitability (Woolf 1983). Previously, it was believed that the hypersensitivity following tissue injury was due to increased excitability of peripheral neurons. However, since tissue damage often has bilateral effects, the underlying mechanisms cannot be purely peripheral. Nowadays, it is known that central sensitization is the main culprit for many of the

1

temporal, spatial and threshold changes seen in both acute and chronic pain stages (Latremoliere & Woolf 2009). However, today, there exists no valid method of quantifying the degree of central sensitization in patients.

In order to investigate and quantify this central sensitization, a novel technique based on the human Nociceptive Withdrawal Reflex (NWR) has been proposed (Andersen 2007; Neziri et al. 2009; Schouenborg et al. 1995; Skljarevski & Ramadan 2002). Since the human NWR is a spinal reflex, conveyed via neurons in the spinal cord, any hypersensitivity in the spinal cord will cause the reflex patterns to change and by using the NWR to quantify these changes, it may be possible to quantify the degree of central sensitization. Being able to assess and quantify the presence of central sensitization will allow clinicians to provide better pain treatment.

1.1 The Nociceptive Withdrawal Reflex

The withdrawal reflex was originally discovered and described by Nobel Prize recipient Sir Charles Sherrington more than a century ago (Sherrington 1910). He referred to the reflex as the flexor reflex as he believed that the reflex occurs by flexing one or more proximal joints to withdraw the limb from a distal noxious stimulation. In these studies both mechanical and electrical stimulations were used to elicit the reflexes. To monitor the evoked reflexes, Sherrington used myographs and photographic kinetoscope analysis. Sherrington also studied the reflex using both decerebrate and intact animal preparations (cats and dogs) and found that similar reflexes could be evoked in both decerebrate and intact preparations indicating a spinal reflex. Since Sherringtons work, the reflex has been the base for substantial research in both humans (Andersen 2007; Hagbarth 1960; Neziri et al. 2010; Rhudy & France 2007; Skljarevski & Ramadan 2002) and animals (Le et al. 2001; Schouenborg et al. 1995). Experimentally, the reflex is typically evoked using electrical stimulation of either an afferent nerve trunk or directly to the skin. However, other stimulation modalities, such as laser stimulation, can also be used to evoke the reflex, but found less synchronized withdrawal patterns than when using electrical stimulation (Morch et al. 2007). The reflex is typically recorded using standard electromyography (EMG).

Today, most researchers use the term the nociceptive withdrawal reflex (NWR) when referring to the evoked physiological response (Andersen 2007; Neziri et al. 2010; Perrotta et al. 2012). The NWR will ensure that any limb, exposed to a noxious stimulus, will be withdrawn optimally from the stimulus to prevent tissue damage. The NWR is a polysynaptic reflex which is mediated through small sensory afferents into the spinal cord where one or more spinal inter-neurons are intercalated in the reflex arc before the motor neurons are activated. When the action potential of the efferent neuron(s) reaches the muscle(s), the muscle(s) will contract and this will mechanically remove the limb from the noxious stimulus (figure 1). The background for renaming the reflex to NWR was that, half a century ago, Hagbarth discovered that the human withdrawal reflex was not solely a flexor reflex but the reflex could also cause the extension of joints (Hagbarth 1960). Furthermore, Hagbarth observed that each reflex will not only cause the contraction of some muscles but will also inhibit other muscles, typically the antagonists of the contracted muscle(s). He hypothesized that the extensor reflexes could be elicited from skin areas covering extensor muscles. Using electrical stimulation in the sole of the human foot, a later study showed that the further distal the stimulation was delivered, the higher tendency to dorsal flexion – by moving the stimulation towards the heel and proximal part of the sole, the tendency to plantar flex (functional extension of the ankle) would be increased (Grimby 1963). The dorsal flexion was consistent with contraction of the Tibialis Anterior (TA) muscle and the plantar flexion was consistent with contraction of Gastrocnemius (GM) and Soleus (SOL) muscles (Grimby 1963). Similarly, Hagbarth found reciprocity between TA and GM muscles, meaning that activation of one would cause inhibition of the other. Grimby also found that reflexes in TA had lower thresholds than those in GM and SOL (Grimby 1963). The findings by Hagbarth and Grimby were elaborated and it was discovered that the NWR had a modular organization. This was first described in rats (Schouenborg & Kalliomaki 1990) and later in man (Andersen et al. 1999). This organization means that stimulation of a certain skin area will only elicit reflexes in a certain muscle or group of synergistic muscles, which, by their contraction, will withdraw the stimulated skin area away from the stimulation. Based on the principle of modular NWR organization a reflex receptive field (RRF) can be mapped for each muscle. It should be noted that some RRFs overlap (Andersen et al. 2005).

The withdrawal patterns of the human upper limbs are quite complex, and are somewhat different to those in the front limbs of animals. Instead, the withdrawal of the legs is simpler and has more resemblance to that of the hind limbs in animals. Thus, the NWR is most often studied in the legs of humans or in the hind limbs in animal preparations (Andersen 2007;

Schouenborg et al. 1995). Studies in humans typically apply electrical stimulation in the sole of the foot or to a nerve trunk at the ankle. One study found that the stimulation even at the dorsum of the foot could evoke NWRs which also showed a modular organization, however, the reflexes were on average 5 times smaller than those elicited from the sole of the foot (Sonnenborg et al. 2001).

Several studies have investigated the spatial organization of the RRFs in the human sole of the foot (Andersen et al. 1999; Andersen et al. 2003; Andersen 2007). Generally, the RRF of each muscle is located in the area which will be withdrawn by that muscle. However, several muscles possess a bi-functionality i.e. besides working as a flexor or extensor they may also function as an inverter or everter. An example of this bi-functionality is the SOL muscle, which has been shown to have two RRFs in the sole of the foot. One RRF was in the heel as would be expected, since SOL is mainly a plantar flexor. However, SOL also have a RRF in the medial arch of the foot (Andersen et al. 1999), this represents SOLs bi-functionality as an inverter (Andersen et al. 1999). Usually, the foci of the RRF are the most sensitive areas and the reflex sensitivity in the RRF decreases towards the borders of the RRF. RRF studies usually focus on the main ankle flexors and extensors but also the knee flexors and extensors. It has been found that the RRF of the more proximal knee muscles will generally cover the entire sole of the foot and the activity in these muscles depends less on the stimulation site (Andersen et al. 2001). Thus, any modular organization of these muscles appears to be less pronounced. A similar finding has been made when stimulating the dorsum of the foot (Sonnenborg et al. 2001). In contrast, the muscles affecting the ankle joint have been found to have more well-defined RRFs. Of these ankle muscles, particularly TA, GM, and SOL have been studied. The RRFs of antagonist muscles overlap (Andersen et al. 2005; Schouenborg & Kalliomaki 1990; Sonnenborg et al. 2001). Thus, the actual functional movement is the sum of the forces generated in the contracted muscles (Andersen et al. 2005). Early studies reported difficulties establishing the exact borders between the inhibitory and excitatory fields (Hagbarth 1960), however, more recent animal studies suggest that these boundaries are in fact well-defined (Schouenborg & Weng 1994). Even so, the resulting movement remains the sum of the forces generated in the contracted muscles (Andersen et al. 2005; Schouenborg & Weng 1994).

In order to distinguish between the NWR and other muscle activity the literature generally suggests to use the reflex latency to determine the origin of the EMG signals (Andersen et al. 1999; Rhudy & France 2007; Terry et al. 2011). Reflexes mediated by faster non-nociceptive Aβ fibers have shorter latencies due to a faster conduction velocity in the afferent fibers, this reflex is also referred to as the RII reflex (Hugon 1973). The NWR, also known as the RIII reflex, is mediated by nociceptive Aδ fibers which have slower conduction velocities than Aβ fibers. Furthermore, voluntary contraction following stimulation could resemble a reflex when seen in the EMG signals. However, such activity will not be of purely spinal origin and must therefore pass through supraspinal centers. This longer conduction pathway will increase the latency and can therefore also be excluded using appropriate latency intervals. Different authors recommend different analysis intervals, however, there seems to be some agreement that the reflex will only be present in the post stimulus interval 60-180 ms after stimulation onset. Obviously, it should be noted that the conduction pathway is somewhat proportional to the height of the subject/patient, hence taller persons will have longer conduction distances and thus longer latencies. Within the reflex window, both a short and long loop reflex have been defined (Andersen et al. 1999) and typically the dorsal flexors exhibited reflexes in the short interval and especially the SOL reflexes exhibited more reflexes in the long loop interval. The longer reflex loop for SOL reflexes evoked at the heel may indicate that these reflexes may be under supra-spinal influence – functionally a valid concept, so if the heel is weight bearing, the ankle is not suddenly plantar flexed as this may cause a fall, potentially inducing an even greater risk of injury.

The strong modular organization of NWRs found using electrical stimulation (Andersen et al. 1999; Andersen 2007), appears to be less prominent for other stimulation modalities (Morch et al. 2007). Furthermore, the reflexes elicited from the sole of the foot are larger than those elicited from the dorsum of the foot. Finally, the withdrawal patterns in the leg are less complicated compared to the arms (Floeter et al. 1998). Therefore, this PhD thesis will focus on reflexes elicited by cutaneous electrical stimulation in the sole of the foot, as done in most of the existing literature based on human RRF studies.

1.1.1 Using the NWR to diagnose central sensitization

The idea to use the NWR as a measure for central sensitization relies greatly on the technique to assess the RRFs. A recent study has shown that the RRFs will expand during chronic pain caused by central sensitization

(Skljarevski & Ramadan 2002). Furthermore, studies have also shown that repetitive painful stimulation will also cause the RRF to expand (Andersen et al. 2005). By comparing the RRFs of patients suffering from chronic pain to normative values (Neziri et al. 2010); researchers hope to be able to determine whether the patients RRF is enlarged, and if that is case, estimate to what degree the patient suffers from central sensitization. Therefore, the NWR appears to be a unique method to non-invasively probe the central nervous system for central sensitization in chronic pain patients.

However, the use of the NWR to probe for central sensitization is only as good as the basic methods for data acquisition and data analysis. It remains somewhat uninvestigated and undocumented that the basic methodology used to elicit and record the NWR are the most optimal methods. Many studies have focused on the analysis and quantification of the NWR (Neziri et al. 2009; Rhudy & France 2007), and how to best quantify the RRFs (Manresa et al. 2011). Instead, this PhD thesis has focused more on the basic methodology, meaning the possibilities for improving NWR elicitation and recording. Any improvement of the basic NWR methodology is highly relevant since the variability of the method, is one of the main factors that prevent it from being routinely used in the clinic.

Aims

The NWR has great potential to be used in clinical and experimental neurophysiology. This PhD project investigated the quality of the standard methodology used to elicit and record the NWR. During the project the following research aims were investigated:

- Is the current method of recording the reflexes prone to EMG crosstalk?
- What factors affect the sensitivity and specificity of the reflex recording? What is the optimal tradeoff between sensitivity and specificity?
- Does afferent input to the CNS vary depending on stimulation site?
- Does skin thickness affect the neuronal activation in the sole of the foot?
- Does the nociceptive innervation vary across the sole of the foot?

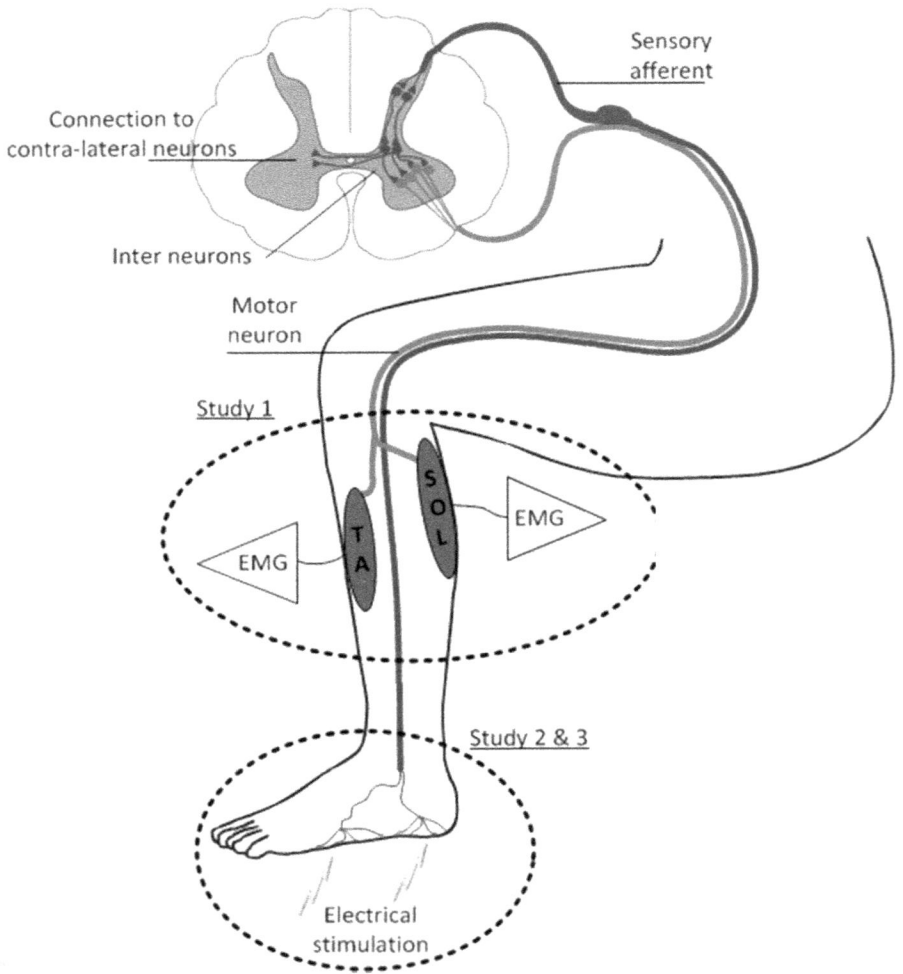

Figure 1. The basic physiology of the NWR and focus points for the studies in this thesis. The shown physiology of the reflex is simplified as the interneurons in the spinal cord are subject to supra spinal modulation. The figure depicts a simplification of the cutaneous nerves innervation in the sole of the foot.

2.1 Overview of study aims

This PhD thesis contains three sub-studies (*I*, *II*, and *III*) each focusing on different aspects of the methodology of the NWR elicitation and recording. Figure 1 depicts how the three studies are linked to the basic neurophysiology of the NWR.

Study I focused on the recording of the NWR using surface EMG. The main problem of recording the reflex is to ensure high sensitivity and high specificity. High sensitivity will ensure that all reflexes will be recorded and not only those sweeps containing larger reflexes. High specificity will ensure that only sweeps containing reflexes are accepted as sweeps containing reflexes. High sensitivity and specificity is needed for the RRFs to be calculated correctly. The primary aim of study I was to document that crosstalk is present in standard NWR recordings using surface electrodes, and investigated different strategies to eliminate or reduce crosstalk.

Study II documented potential problems concerning reflex elicitation from the sole of the foot related to activation of Aδ fiber nociceptors. Several studies have reported difficulties evoking reflexes from the heel and that the use of much higher stimulation intensities were required to evoke reflexes from the heel (Andersen et al. 1999). However, differences in neural activation when stimulating the sole of the foot in humans have never been documented in detail. Therefore, the aim of *study II* was primarily to investigate and document the apparent differences in neural activation across the sole. Secondly, to develop a model to investigate how differences in the volume conductor, primarily caused by thicker skin at the heel and pads, can explain the differences in the neural activation.

Study III investigated the nociceptive innervation in the sole of the foot and applied advanced neural modeling to investigate differences in afferent activity associated with different stimulation sites. In *study II* it was assumed that the nociceptive innervation in humans across the sole of the foot is not site dependent. However, this has never been documented previously. Only the mechanoreceptors have previously been mapped (Kennedy & Inglis 2002). Therefore, the primary aims in *study III* were to stain the nociceptive innervation in the sole of the foot and secondly to apply more advanced neural modeling to investigate if the activation thresholds of Aδ and Aβ are site dependent.

1.2 Papers

Study I
Surface EMG crosstalk during phasic involuntary muscle activation in the nociceptive withdrawal reflex.
KS Frahm, MB Jensen, D Farina, OK Andersen. Muscle Nerve **46**: 228–236, 2012

Study II
Experimental and model-based analysis of differences in perception of cutaneous electrical stimulation across the sole of the foot.
KS Frahm, CD Mørch, WM Grill, OK Andersen. Med Biol Eng Comput. **51**: 999-1009, 2013

Study III
Activation of peripheral nerve fibers by electrical stimulation in the sole of the foot.
KS Frahm, CD Mørch, WM Grill, NB Lubock, K Hennings, OK Andersen. BMC Neuroscience **14**:116, 2013

Methods

This chapter will discuss the methods applied in this PhD thesis. For ***study I*** primarily the EMG techniques and analysis of these signals will be discussed. For ***study II*** the psychophysical evaluation methods and modeling techniques will be discussed. For ***study III*** the staining techniques and advanced neural modeling will be discussed.

3.1 Reflex monitoring (study I)

In order to map the RRF, it is critical to determine which stimulation sites a muscle(s) can be activated from. As mentioned above, the standard method for recording reflexes is by surface EMG (sEMG). However, it can often be difficult to know exactly which muscle is activated since all biological tissue acts as a volume conductor and thus sEMG can be recorded even if the electrodes are not placed immediately adjacent to the active muscle (Farina et al. 2004b). This phenomenon is known as crosstalk and is a problem occurring in many sEMG recordings, e.g. a reflex in the TA muscle can be recorded via electrodes placed on top of the SOL muscle. sEMG signals prone to crosstalk will have reduced specificity and considering how the RRFs are mapped, crosstalk obviously will pose a problem and, to a degree, create incorrect RRFs, further limiting the NWR/RRF usability to probe for central sensitization. Alternatively, other modalities like goniometer or accelerometers have been used to monitor reflexes in conjunction with EMG (Andersen et al. 1999; Andersen et al. 2005; Sonnenborg et al. 2001). However, unlike EMG, goniometers and accelerometers measure the resultant joint movement based on all muscle activity in the limb and not the activity of each muscle, making it impossible to determine the RRF of single muscles. Furthermore, in case of small reflexes, where the resulting net movement is small, goniometers and accelerometer may not have sufficiently high sensitivity to register the reflex. Since the assessment of the RRF is critical when determining the degree of central sensitization, the reflexes in the thesis were assessed using EMG. The main challenge of sEMG acquisition remains to ensure high specificity – meaning reducing crosstalk in the sEMG recordings.

3.1.1 Electromyography

Several methods to reduce or eliminate crosstalk have been suggested; however, many of these methods have later been rejected. Since the crosstalk is volume conducted through the tissue, this may create a signal with lower frequency components than genuine EMG signals. Therefore, it was hypothesized to use high-pass (HP) filtering to eliminate crosstalk. However, this hypothesis has been rejected, since studies have shown that crosstalk can contain more high-frequency components than genuine muscle signals (Farina et al. 2004b). The origin of the high frequent components is related to generation of the crosstalk signals occurring at the end-plates of muscles (Farina et al. 2004b). Use of cross-correlation analysis has also been suggested to distinguish crosstalk from genuine muscle signals. However, this method is not valid since the volume conductor changes the phase of the signal and not only the magnitude of the signal (De Luca & Merletti 1988; Farina et al. 2002). Instead, spatial filtering of EMG has been suggested for further crosstalk reduction (Farina 2006) e.g. the use of double differential (DD) recording instead of single differential (SD) or by using shorter inter electrode distance (IED).

To compare different recording parameters and evaluate how the crosstalk and sensitivity was affected three modalities of EMG recordings were used to record reflexes (figure 2): single channel surface-EMG (sEMG), multi-channel sEMG and intramuscular EMG (iEMG). In most prior studies, sEMG has been the standard method to record reflexes (Sandrini et al. 2005; Skljarevski & Ramadan 2002). Both a SD and DD were used in the single-channel setup (DD setup not illustrated in figure 2). A 1x8 electrode array was recorded as 7 channels of SD sEMG (multi-channel) to enable an offline analysis of different IEDs for both SD and DD. iEMG has the advantage of being almost completely unaffected by crosstalk (van Vugt & van Dijk 2001) (figure 2) – however, as the name indicates, either a needle or wire has to be inserted into the muscle. The insertion of the iEMG electrode will undoubtly be associated with discomfort for the subject/patient and a larger infection risk. Typically, iEMG has very small pickup area and will only record from few motor units. This means that a reflex in a muscle might not be recorded if the reflex only involves activity in few motor units. In order to overcome this problem and obtain a more general *gross* muscle EMG the used fine wire had the insulation removed 5 mm from the tip. This allowed a larger pick-up area, and thus recording from more motor units. The electrode setup can be seen in figure 3.

Type	Example	Pros	Cons	Impedance
sEMG				
Single channel	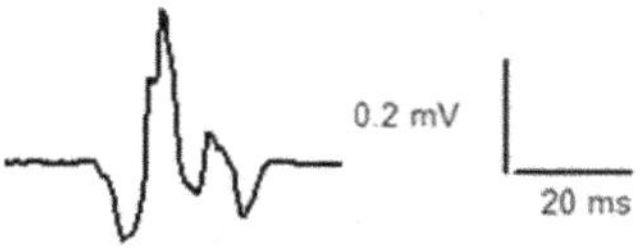 0.2 mV / 20 ms	High sensitivity, easy mounting	Low selectivity	Low
Multi channel	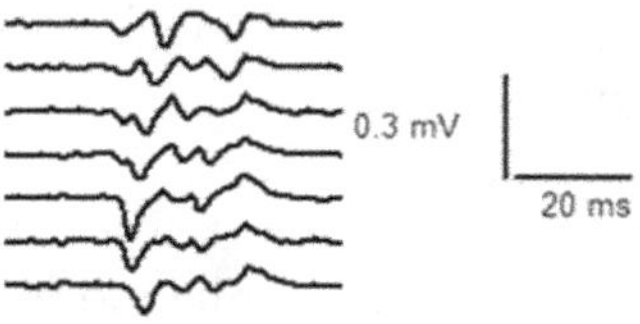 0.3 mV / 20 ms	Medium selectivity, possible to see travelling MU-AP	Low sensitivity, Single channel, difficult to mount	Medium
iEMG	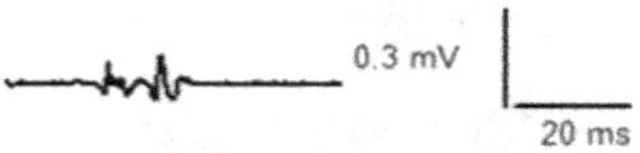 0.3 mV / 20 ms	No crosstalk, medium sensitivity	Bleeding, infection, discomfort, no gross muscle EMG, difficult to mount	High

Figure 2. Overview of different EMG electrode setups used in *study I*. The single channel sEMG recordings refer to the use of Ambu Neuroline 720 electrodes. The multi-channel refers to the use of the 1x8 array electrodes. The examples are actual recordings from *study I*. All recordings shown here are recorded using a single differential setup.

To quantify the crosstalk, a RMS z-score was calculated as the primary analysis. The RMS z-score was defined as the difference between the RMS of the reflex window 60 to 180 ms post stimulation onset and RMS of 120 ms baseline, divided with the standard deviation of the 120 ms baseline. The RMS z-score was calculated both for the agonist and antagonist muscles. Besides the RMS z-score, an algorithm for reflex detection (France et al. 2009; Rhudy & France 2007) was also used. The reflex detection algorithm would reveal how well the use of e.g. DD will be effective for either detecting or discarding reflexes in EMG recordings. Furthermore, cross-correlation of the enveloped signal was calculated between the agonist iEMG and antagonist SD sEMG and DD sEMG, respectively. The cross-correlation analysis was applied to test whether the DD recordings, besides reducing the magnitude of the crosstalk, could also affect the correlation of the crosstalk signal compared to the genuine muscle signal.

Since only the ankle flexors and extensors have localized RRFs restricted to the sole of the foot, only these muscles were monitored to study the EMG. To monitor EMG from dorsal flexors, TA was chosen as the primary dorsal flexor as used in several previous studies (Andersen et al. 1999; Sonnenborg et al. 2000). The main plantar flexor is the triceps surae group (GM, and SOL), but since GM are biarticular muscles, causing both ankle *and* knee flexion, *study I* focused on SOL.

Previous studies investigating methods for reducing crosstalk in EMG signals used efferent nerve stimulation to elicit the muscle activity (De Luca & Merletti 1988; Farina et al. 2002). However, this approach results in unnatural activation of motor units and thus it was necessary to test whether the findings of these studies could be applied to NWR recordings associated with natural motor unit recruitment. Thus, to evoke EMG activity, electrical stimulation was applied in the sole of the foot.

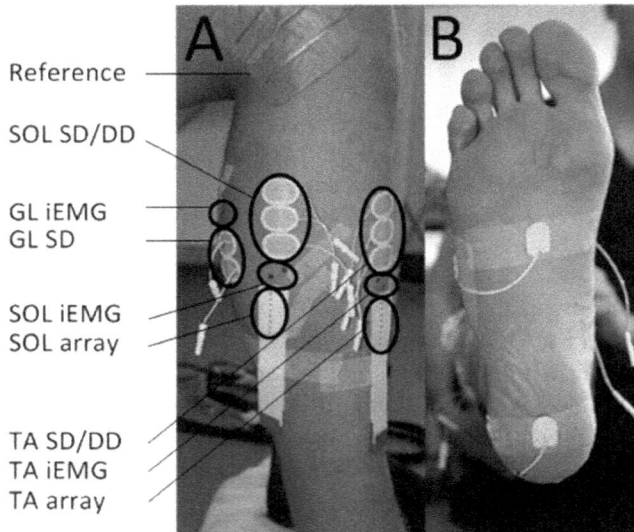

Figure 3. The electrode configurations used in *study I* for EMG recording (A) and stimulation (B). The reference used for stimulation is not visible in (B), but was placed on the dorsum of the foot. The EMG setups for TA and SOL were identical. Furthermore, GL was monitored for any contraction with SOL to ensure that any activity in the SOL EMG did not originate from the GL muscle (crosstalk). Note that the single channel electrodes for both TA and SOL were used for both SD and DD recording.

3.2 Noxious stimulation (study I & II)

Elicitation of the NWR occurs due to the activation of a sufficient amount of cutaneous nociceptors to any form of noxious stimuli. Experimentally, the reflex is mostly evoked using electrical stimulation, even though thermal stimuli have also been used in humans (Morch et al. 2007) – and mechanical stimuli have been used in animal preparations (Sherrington 1910). The problem with both mechanical and thermal stimuli is that the stimulus duration is quite a bit longer than those needed when employing electrical stimulation (200 ms (Morch et al. 2007) vs. 25 ms (Andersen et al. 1999)). Since the reflex window is calculated to a maximum window until 180 ms after stimulus onset a longer latency may overlap the reflex window – 60 to 180 ms post stimulus. In fact when using thermal stimulus the evoked reflexes was less synchronized than when using electrical stimulation (Morch et al. 2007). Therefore, electrical stimulation appears to be the most optimal technique to elicit NWRs in order to map the RRF.

The stimulation paradigm for the electrical stimulation has previously been investigated, and it was found that a train of five 1 ms pulses delivered at 200 Hz is most effective for eliciting reflexes (Tørring et al. 1981). This is good agreement with the fact that sensory neurons have lower activation thresholds than motor neurons for electrical pulses longer than 0.5 ms (Panizza et al. 1998). Since the NWR is evoked by sensory afferents, and co-activation of motor fibers is unwanted, this it is further evidence that paradigm suggested by (Tørring et al. 1981) is optimal to elicit NWRs. Therefore, this method (Tørring et al. 1981) was used to stimulate the sole for reflex elicitation (*study I*) and to map the neural activation in the sole (*study II*). However, the purpose of *study II* was to get a more geographical information of the variation of the neural activation, therefore six stimulation site were used instead of two (figure 4).

In *study I* and *II* the stimulating electrodes were placed in the sole of the foot (Neuroline 700, Ambu, Denmark) (figures 3 & 4), and a larger electrode 10 x 7 cm placed on the dorsum served as the reference (Pals, Axelgaard, USA). In *study I*, the stimulation intensity was normalized as 1.5 times the NWR threshold. The threshold was defined as the minimal intensity that evoked at least two reflexes in three stimulations. In case of habituation causing the reflex to disappear, the threshold was reevaluated. To elicit reflexes in TA, stimulation was delivered in the focus of the TA RRF, meaning the medial arch in the sole of the foot (figures 3 & 4A). To elicit reflexes in SOL, stimulation was delivered at the heel (figure 3 & 4A).

In *study II*, the stimulation intensity was normalized to the perception threshold. The perception threshold was identified using a staircase method involving three ascending and three descending staircases. Stimulation intensities of 2x and 4x perception threshold were subsequently used. At each of the six sites, three different electrode sizes were tested, to identify to what degree the neural activation changed for graded electrode size.

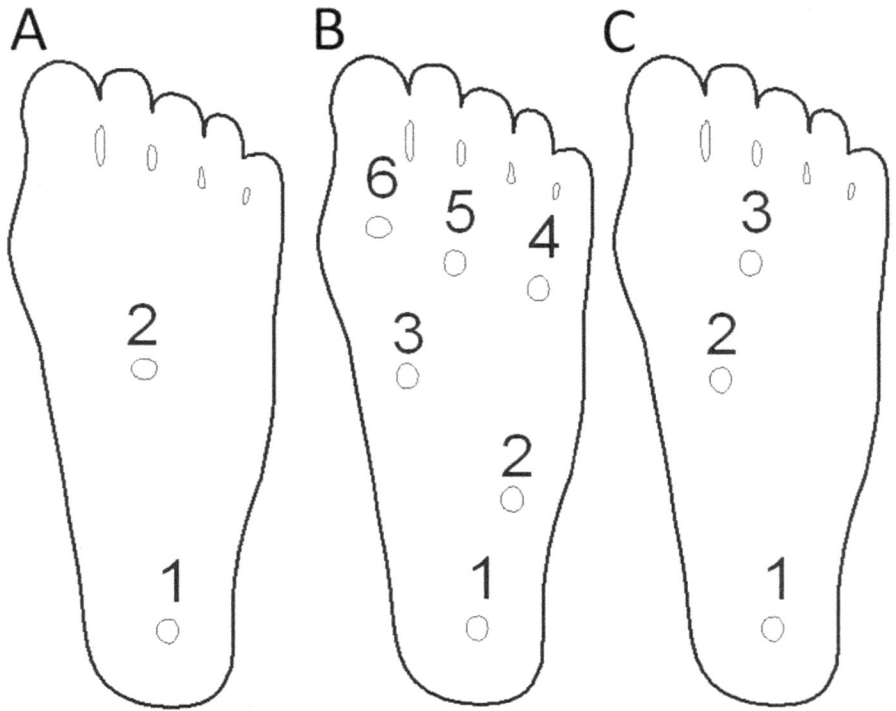

Figure 4. The sites used in *study I*, *II* and *III*. A) In *study I*, electrical stimulation was applied in the arch of foot to elicit reflexes in TA, or in the heel of the foot to elicit reflexes in SOL. B) In *study II*, six sites were stimulated, modeled, and measured using ultrasound scans and skin biopsies. In *study II*, site 1 was the heel, site 2 was the lateral arch, site 3 was the medial arch, site 4, 5, and 6 were the underneath the lateral, central and medial metatarsals, respectively. C) In *study III*, three sites were modeled and stained for nerves. Sites 1, 3, and 5 from *study II* were identical with sites 1, 2, and 3 from *study III*, respectively.

3.3 Mapping the neural activation in the sole of the foot (study II)

In order to determine whether the neural activation depends on the stimulation site, a number of different approaches can be used. The neural activation of interest was primarily the activation of the Aδ fibers. Since different afferent fiber types have different conduction velocities, EMG or EEG analysis may rely on the timing of the recorded compound action potentials to differentiate between fiber types. However, the intensity of the neural activation can be difficult to deduct directly from the EMG/EEG or similar measures. Instead verbal measures like pain questionnaires can be used.

3.3.1 Pain questionnaires

It is well established that the perceived quality of any cutaneous stimulation reflects the type of afferent fiber activated (Gracely 1999). Previous studies have investigated the sensory input from electrical stimulation using a pain quality questionnaire (Hansen et al. 2007; Morch et al. 2011). One of the used questionnaires (Hansen et al. 2007) is in German, which limits the use to German-speaking subjects. However, other questionnaires exist, such as the McGill Pain Questionnaire (MPQ) (Melzack 1975), which was used in (Morch et al. 2011). The MPQ is in English and has been translated and validated in multiple languages (Drewes et al. 1993; Maiani & Sanavio 1985). The MPQ was designed to be used when gathering the anamnesis of a new patient, and only to be filled out once by the patient or subject. The questionnaire contains 20 groups of descriptors with several sub-descriptors in each group making it unfeasible to use with multiple combinations of stimulus parameters such as stimulus site and electrode size. Furthermore, the questionnaire contains sensory, affective, and evaluative descriptors, where the latter two does not give any information about the type of fiber activated. Instead, it was necessary to use a measure which the subjects could easily grasp and quickly rate. For this purpose the full size MPQ is too cumbersome to use and would require too much work from the subjects. Instead, the MPQ has been revised into a short-form version (SF-MPQ) (Melzack 1987) containing less descriptive groups. The SF-MPQ contains 11 sensory descriptors and 4 affective descriptors. Each of these 15 descriptors is rated as either None, Mild, Moderate or Severe. Since the study was only focused on the type of sensory fibers activated, only the 11 sensory groups were presented to the subjects. Finally, as a measure of the intensity of the stimulations, the Visual Analog Scale (VAS) was presented to the subjects along with the SF-MPQ. The VAS score is a standard tool used in pain research as a measure of pain intensity (Gracely 1999) and often used in conjunction with both the MPQ and SF-MPQ (Melzack 1987). The VAS score used in this thesis was anchored as 0 – No pain and 10 – Worst Imaginable pain.

3.4 Volume conductor modeling (study II & III)

Mathematical modeling was applied to investigate the differences in neural activation at different sites. There is no doubt that the skin thicknesses vary substantially across the sole of the foot, especially the skin at the heel and pads is much thicker than in the arch. Differences in skin composition and thicknesses may alter the volume conduction through the tissue. One way to investigate the differences is to establish a computer model using the finite element method (FEM) to model the volume conduction through the tissue. This will allow estimation of how variation in skin thickness and other tissue types affect the current flow in the tissue. The FEM enables the easy use of more advanced model geometries and easy implementation of both resistive and capacitive components. The downside is the need for substantial more computational power than if using analytical models.

3.4.1 The finite element method

To model the current density distribution in the tissue the software package from COMSOL Multiphysics (Stockholm, Sweden) was used. The model was designed using rotational symmetry (figure 5). This was done to limit the computational burden, making it more feasible to run the same model a number of times to test different parameters like electrode size, stimulation site etc. The model comprised seven tissue types; the stratum corneum, vital epidermis, dermis, fat layer, muscle tissue, cortical bone and bone marrow (figure 5). The geometry was based on ultrasound scans from healthy subjects and skin biopsies from post-mortem feet. The geometry design was simplified and does not in detail represent the placement of the stimulation electrode and reference electrode. The electrical properties incorporated both resistive and capacitive elements of the tissues using a di-electrical model. Evidently, the model effectively showed that current conduction through the tissue changed slightly during the course of a constant current stimulation as expected due to capacitive effects.

In *study II* all tissues were modeled as being isotropic, but since *study III* was especially focused on modeling neural tissues located in vital layers of the skin (dermis and vital epidermis), it was necessary to include a more accurate description of the electrical properties of these layers; for instance it is well known that the epidermis and dermis are highly anisotropic tissues (Tavernier et al. 1993). The inclusion of anisotropic properties for both the vital epidermis and dermis leads to a more precise description of the extracellular potential to be used in conjunction with the neural model.

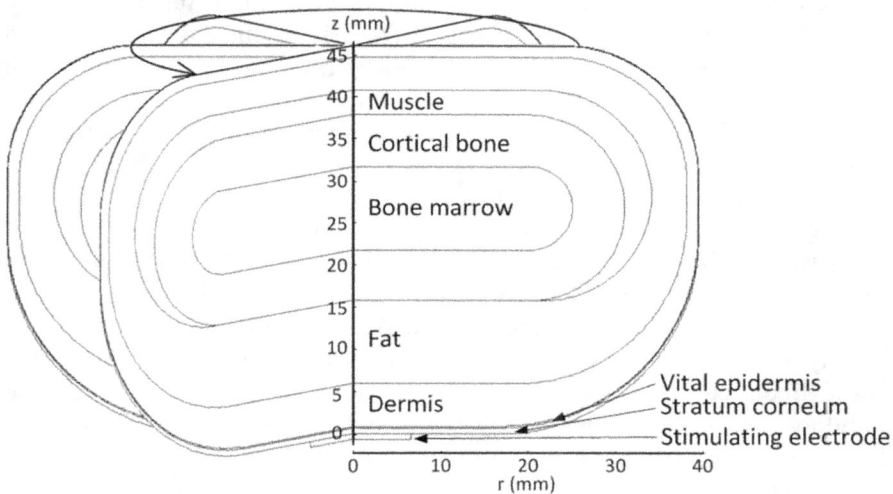

Figure 5. The geometry of the finite element model used in *study II* and *III*. The model comprised seven different tissue types as indicated in the figure. The geometry of the model was adjusted according to stimulation site. The depicted geometry corresponds to site 1, the heel.

3.5 Estimations of nerve activation (study II & III)

Since Hodgkin and Huxley's work (Hodgkin & Huxley 1952) many models have been developed to describe the generation and conduction of action potentials (AP) in neurons e.g. (Grill 1999; McNeal 1976; Rattay

1986; Reilly et al. 1985). When reviewing the literature it seems that most studies have focused on modeling larger myelinated motor neurons. Little focus has been directed towards investigating thinly myelinated and unmyelinated afferents, like those found in the skin. The complexity of previous models varies from simple (Rattay 1986) to highly complex models incorporating accurate representation of the electrical properties of the myelin layer and representation of the different ion channels found in the node of Ranvier and paranodal areas (McIntyre et al. 2002).

In *study II* the main focus of the modeling was the volume conductor. The different skin thickness across the sole would undoubtedly change the volume conductor. Therefore, it was relevant to combine a simple estimate for the neural activation with the FEM, e.g. the activation function (Rattay 1986). Basically the activation function (AF) is calculated as the second derivative of the extracellular potential oriented along the direction of the nerve fibers, i.e. for most cutaneous afferents, perpendicular to the skin surface. Combining the volume conductor model with the activation function was intended to give an overview of how the activation of nerves would change due to differences in the volume conductor.

In *study III* the FEM was slightly updated as indicated above, but the main focus was on the neural model. The desired outcome of the model was to determine whether activation of the cutaneous afferents differed across the sole. Since the NWR is mediated by Aδ fibers the model focused on this fiber type, however, the electrical stimulation may also activate Aβ fibers. These fibers can also elicit RII reflexes with a shorter latency than the withdrawal reflexes (Hugon 1973). Furthermore, the perception threshold during electrical stimulation is normally correlated to the Aβ activation threshold (Hugon 1973), unless extremely small electrodes are used (Morch et al. 2011). Thus, in order to compare the model to both perception threshold and pain threshold, both Aδ and Aβ fibers were modeled using a simplified version of the McNeal model (McNeal 1976). By leaving out the capacitive term in the model, it was possible to model realistic representations of the density of the nerves found in the skin. The model was used to describe how the trans-membrane potential would change in presence of extracellular potentials along the nerve fiber. When the trans-membrane potential of the fibers had been depolarized by 20 mV or more, it was assumed that an AP would be initiated. Obviously, it should be noted that activation of a single afferent nerve fibers is insufficient to evoke reflexes or any kind of perception.

To make sure that both the volume conductor and nerve models had realistic representations of the tissue geometries, a series of anatomical studies were performed prior to computer modeling. Furthermore, without knowledge of the innervation density all modeling would have to assume similar innervation across the sole of the foot; however, this has not been proven in detail. Therefore, to ensure the model incorporated realistic values of the nerve innervation density, a number of nerve staining studies were made.

3.6 Nerve staining and anatomical studies (study II & III)

A series of anatomical studies were carried out to determine the gross anatomy of the tissue and to determine the presence and density of the cutaneous nerves in the sole of the foot. To determine the tissue geometry preferably non-invasive methods should be used so the measures can be obtained from healthy subjects. However, methods like ultrasound scans do not offer sufficiently high resolution to separate different skin layers. High-resolution ultrasound is capable of separating the epidermis from the dermis, but cannot separate the layers inside the epidermis (Frahm et al. 2010). However, more invasive methods like skin biopsies offer very high resolution of different skin layers, but can be limited with respect to measuring tissues deeper than hypodermis due to their soft consistency causing such tissue to be destroyed more easily. The thickness of stratum corneum (SC) was especially important since it has much lower conductivity than other tissues (Gabriel et al. 1996; Tavernier et al. 1993; Yamamoto & Yamamoto 1976) and, hence, it will have a large effect on the overall volume conductor. In *study II* a combination of skin biopsies and ultrasound scans were used. The skin biopsies gave information concerning the thickness of the SC and vital part of the epidermis; whereas the ultrasound scans provided measures of the entire skin thickness (SC, vital epidermis and dermis combined), the fat layer beneath the dermis and the muscle layer.

3.6.1 Nerve staining techniques

Nerve fibers were stained in *study III* in order to discover any differences in innervation density across the sole of the foot. Many studies have used the PGP9.5 antibody to stain nerves in the skin (Ebenezer et al. 2007; Hilliges et al. 1995; Kennedy & Wendelschafer-Crabb 1993; McCarthy et al. 1995). This antibody is very potent to stain neural tissue; but it will not discriminate between the types of neural tissue.

A recent study showed that four specific sodium channels, Na_v 1.6, 1.7, 1.8 and 1.9 can be found in unmyelinated nerve fibers inside the epidermis (Persson et al. 2010). Studies have also shown that Na_v 1.8 and Na_v 1.9 channels are TTX-resistant channels (Catterall et al. 2005; Dib-Hajj et al. 2009; Hernandez-Plata et al. 2012) while Na_v 1.6 and Na_v 1.7 are TTX sensitive (Catterall et al. 2005; Dib-Hajj et al. 2009; Hernandez-Plata et al. 2012). Usually C-fibers are considered TTX-resistant, and in fact Na_v 1.8 and Na_v 1.9, are found predominately in C-fibers (Tu et al. 2010). Thus, staining for Na_v 1.6 or Na_v 1.7 would include most A-fibers. Person et al (Persson et al. 2010) showed that Na_v 1.6 can be found in approximately 70 % of all intraepidermal fibers, whereas Na_v 1.7 is expressed in 90 %. Furthermore, studies have shown that Na_v 1.7 is highly expressed in small myelinated DRG neurons such as the Aδ fiber, whereas the Na_v 1.6 is mainly expressed in larger myelinated DRG neurons (Aβ) and is mainly expressed at the node of Ranvier (Herzog et al. 2003). However, other studies have shown that Na_v 1.6 can be found in C-fibers (Black et al. 2002). Furthermore, studies have showed expression of Na_v 1.7 and Na_v 1.8 in both dermis and epidermis (Persson et al. 2010). However, a very recent study indicated that besides Aδ expression Na_v1.7 can also be found in C-fibers (Black et al. 2012). Thus, it seems that none of the four sodium subchannels are 100 % specific for Aδ fibers. However, Na_v 1.7 appear to be highly expressed in Aδ (Herzog et al. 2003) – and thus the most suitable target for Aδ staining. Aδ fibers lose their myelin sheath when crossing from dermis into epidermis (Reilly et al. 1997) and therefore, inside the epidermis the Aδ fibers will resemble unmyelinated C-fibers.

Furthermore, deep innervation cannot be seen on skin biopsies as these are only a few millimeters thick. To stain for deeper located nerves, the Sihler whole nerve stain technique was applied. The Sihler technique is not fiber type specific and works by staining the myelin of the nerves. Hence, both Aδ and Aβ fibers will be stained. However, the results of this technique would in combination with the Na_v1.7 thoroughly investigate the innervation of primarily the Aδ fibers in the sole of the foot. The innervation was investigated from three sites in the sole of the foot: the heel, the arch, and the forefoot underneath the central metatarsal (figure 4).

Results

This PhD thesis has focused on the recording and elicitation of the human nociceptive withdrawal reflex. In *study I* 15 healthy male subjects participated in the experiments. In *study II* 8 healthy subjects participated in the electrophysiological experiments and ultrasound scans. For the anatomical studies in *study II* and *III*, two post-mortem feet specimens were used.

4.1 Optimized reflex monitoring (study I)

In order to quantify the effect of the tested electrode size and recording setup the RMS z-score for each reflex was calculated (Frahm et al. 2012). Furthermore, the reflex detection algorithm developed by Rhudy and France (Rhudy & France 2007) was also used to investigate the sensitivity and specificity in the EMG recordings (not published) (figures 6, 7, and 8). Both the RMS z-score and the detection ratio showed that the use of SD recordings compared to DD recording would entail significantly higher levels of crosstalk, meaning DD recordings will improve the specificity of the recordings significantly. Similarly to previous results (Farina et al. 2004a; Mesin et al. 2009), the amount of crosstalk increased with increasing IED and pick-up area. Both findings are not surprising since the sensitivity will increase when increasing IED and pick-up area and thus the specificity is expected to suffer from this. Hence, the optimal recording setup is a tradeoff between high sensitivity and specificity. Since DD recordings work as a spatial filter it was expected to observe lower sensitivity than SD, however, despite significant difference for the multichannel recordings (figure 7 and 8), the multi-channel EMG recordings with IEDs of 15-20 mm detected 92-96 % of all reflexes in the DD recordings from the TA and 64-72 % of all reflexes in the DD recordings from SOL. Furthermore, an IED of 15-20 mm resulted in less than 2 % false detections of TA reflexes detected as SOL reflexes and less than 5 % false detections of SOL reflexes detected as TA reflexes. In addition the DD single-channel EMG had a detection level of more than 95 % for true-positive and less than 50 % false-positive detection (figure 6), this shows the effect of a large pick-up area of the electrodes, which increases the sensitivity but lowers the specificity.

For future reflex recording the use of DD is recommended and to ensure a sufficient high level of sensitivity IEDs of 15-20 mm appear to be optimal while still suppressing unwanted crosstalk. Regarding the pick-up area there needs to be made a choice regarding sensitivity vs. specificity.

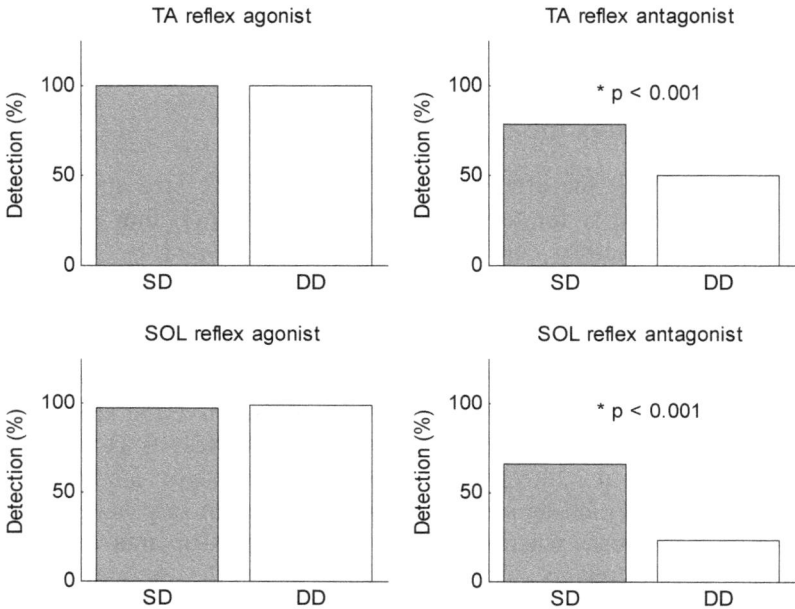

Figure 6. Average ratio of reflex detection – single channel recording. The sensitivity for DD recordings for both TA and SOL was more than 95 % for genuine reflexes. For the TA reflex the DD was capable of reducing the probability of more than 75 % false-positive reflex detection to less than 50 % false-positive reflex detection. For SOL the detection probability was reduced from more than 60 % false-positive reflex detection to less than 25 % false-positive reflex detection. For the genuine muscle signals recorded on the agonist muscle there were minor differences between SD and DD when assessed by the reflex detection algorithm (Rhudy & France 2007). In contrast, the crosstalk signals recorded on top of the antagonist muscle showed significantly higher reflex detection in the SD recordings than the DD, indicating that SD contains significantly more crosstalk than DD. Non-published results.

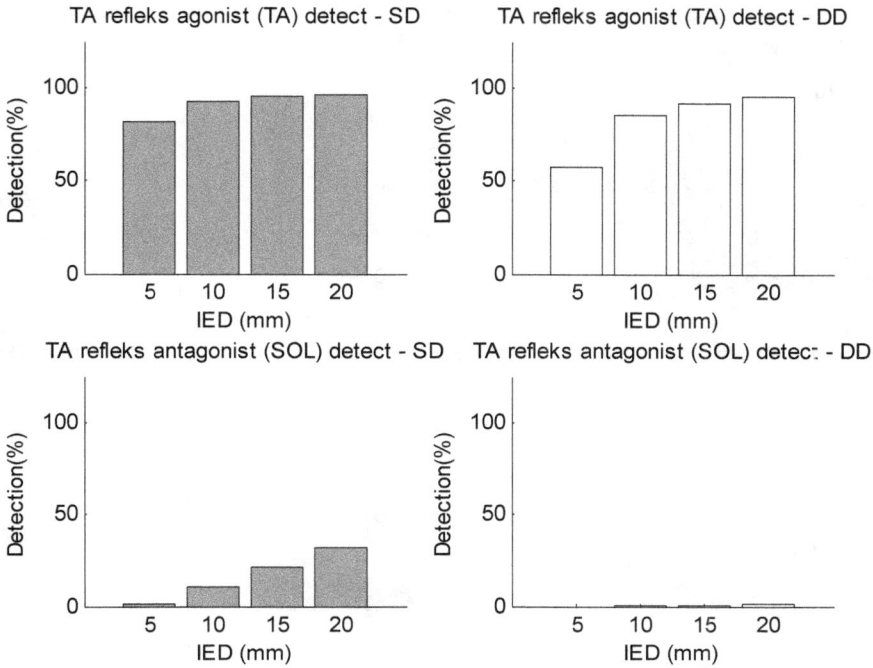

Figure 7. Average ratio of reflex detection for reflexes in TA for varying IEDs – multichannel SD recording. The SD recordings had higher average reflex detection for both agonist (genuine reflexes) and antagonist (crosstalk) than DD (ANOVA, p < 0.001). This means SD recording has higher sensitivity but DD recordings are more selective and less prone to detect crosstalk as reflexes. Based on this data an optimal EMG recording appears to be 15-20 mm DD. IED: inter-electrode-distance. Non-published results.

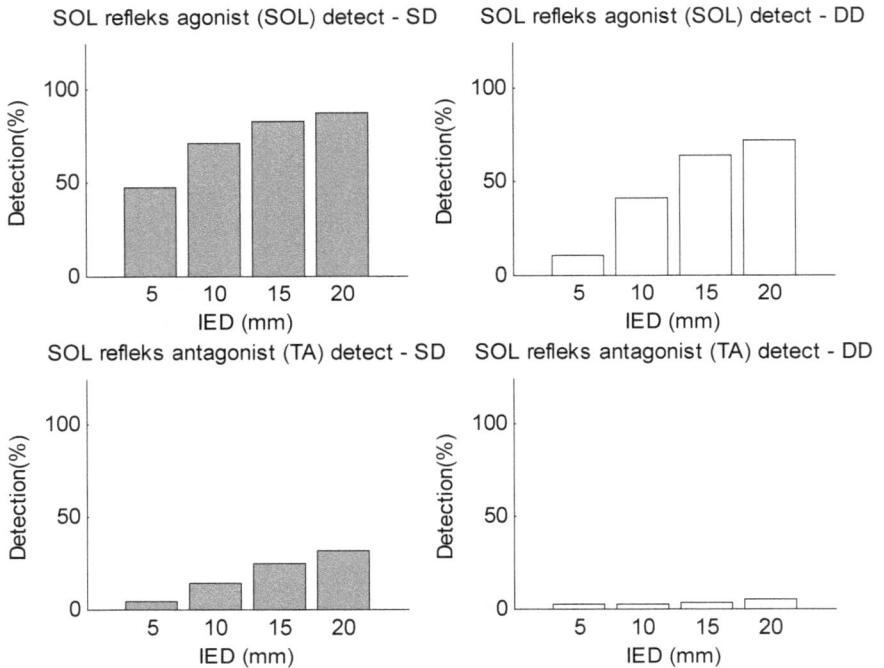

Figure 8. Average ratio of reflex detection during reflexes in SOL for varying IEDs – multi-channel recording. The SD recordings had higher average reflex detection for both agonist (genuine reflexes) and antagonist (crosstalk) than DD (ANOVA, p < 0.001). This means SD recording has higher sensitivity but DD recordings are more selective and less prone to detect crosstalk as reflexes. Based on this data an optimal EMG recording appears to be 15-20 mm DD. IED: inter-electrode-distance. Non-published results.

4.2 Reflex detection and quantification (study I)

Besides the electrode setup, the post-recording data analysis can also support the reduction of crosstalk and help to ensure both high sensitivity and specificity.

In order to automate the detection of reflexes an algorithm to detect the NWR has recently been suggested (France et al. 2009). The detection algorithm is based on deriving the RMS z-score in each EMG sweep, as done in **study I**, and if this value is above 12, then the sweep is defined as containing a reflex. As shown in **study I** the RMS z-score depends greatly on the IED and size of electrode pick-up area (figures 4, 5, and 6 in (Frahm et al. 2012)). Surprisingly, such parameters have *not* been reported by Rhudy and France trying to define this reflex threshold (France et al. 2009; Rhudy & France 2007). Based on the findings in this thesis (figures 6, 7, and 8) it seems that the electrode setup used in (France et al. 2009) had rather small pick-up area, as the best separation of crosstalk is seen in the multi-channel recordings that were acquired using a small pick-up area (10 mm^2). However, this is purely speculative, unfortunately.

Compared to the reflex window (60-180 ms post stimulus) used in this thesis, many other sources suggest using a shorter window to quantify the reflexes (France et al. 2009; Rhudy & France 2007). However, many studies focus on more proximal muscles and elicited by nerve trunk stimulation making the conduction distance shorter than in this case, thus the 60-180 ms post stimulus window appear to be valid to use for reflexes measured in the lower leg evoked by stimulation in the sole of the foot.

4.3 Understanding the neural activation in the sole of the foot (study II & III)

Electrical stimulation in the sole of the foot will cause cutaneous nociceptors to depolarize and thus elicit the NWR if a sufficient amount of nociceptors are activated. Previous results indicate that activation of the NWR is site dependent, indicating that the Aδ fiber activation is site dependent (Andersen et al. 2001). But this has not been documented in detail. Therefore, **study II** attempted to experimentally map the neural activation following electrical stimulation. **Study III** investigated any found differences using advanced neural modeling and nerve stainings.

4.3.1 Experimental map of the Aδ fiber activation in the sole of the foot (study II)

Differences in, what appeared to be Aδ fiber activation, were found between the heel and the other sites, including the arch and forefoot. The McGill questionnaire results found significant differences in the pain descriptors indicating activation of different fiber types. The descriptor *Sharp* is especially interesting since it is known to primarily reflect

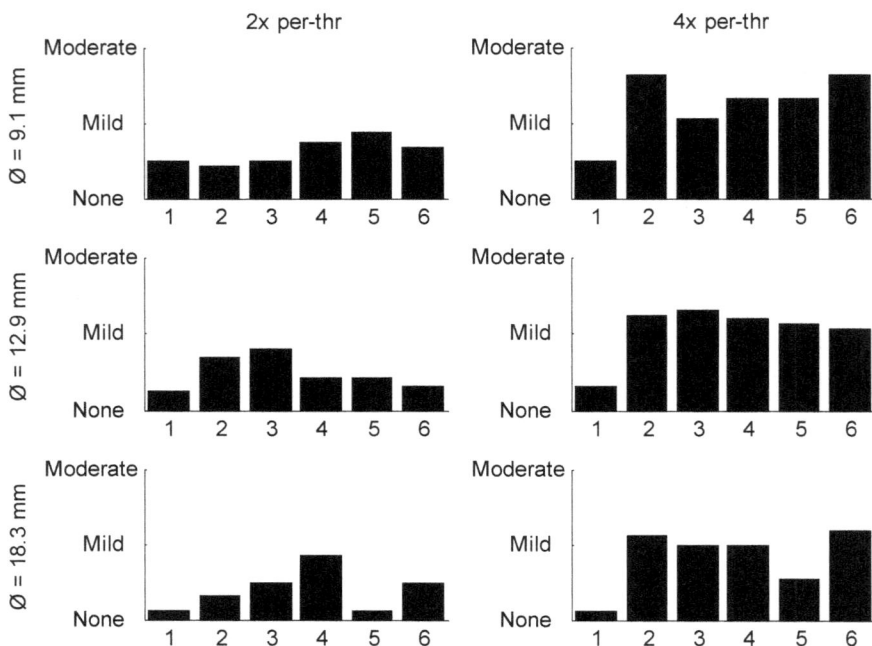

Figure 9. Average distribution of the descriptor *Sharp* on the Short-Form McGill pain questionnaire (SF-MPQ) following stimulation at two and four times the perception threshold (per-thr). The *Sharp* descriptor is the best estimator on the SF-MPQ for the activation of Aδ fibers, mediating the NWR. The intensities of the descriptor were rated as 0: None, 1: Mild, 2: Moderate, 3: Severe. The use of the descriptor *Sharp* was significantly lower at site 1 (the heel) compared to other sites, except site 5. This indicates that electrical stimulation at the heel is less prone to activate Aδ fibers than at the rest of the sole. The ratings were more *sharp* when the size of the electrodes decreased (Log. Reg., $p < 0.05$, Bonferroni corrected). The ratings were significantly more *sharp* for increasing stimulus intensity (Log. Reg., $p < 0.05$, Bonferroni corrected).

activation of Aδ fibers (Hansen et al. 2007). The level of Aδ fiber activation was significantly lower at the heel than all other sites (except site 5) (Log. Reg., $p < 0.05$, Bonferroni corrected, figure 9). Therefore, it seems that electrical stimulation at the heel is less prone to activate Aδ fibers than at the rest of the foot. Despite this apparent lower activation of Aδ fibers, there were found no differences in the perception threshold across the sole of the foot which is in contrast to previous findings (Andersen et al. 2001). This can be due to a higher level of callus removal on the heel than in the study by (Andersen et al. 2001). The heel had higher average detection threshold and lower average VAS scores than the rest of the sole, however, this was not found as significant (figure 10). The findings of lower $A\delta$ fiber activation at the heel fit well with previous studies which indicate that reflexes from the heel were either more difficult to evoke or were less synchronized (Andersen et al. 1999).

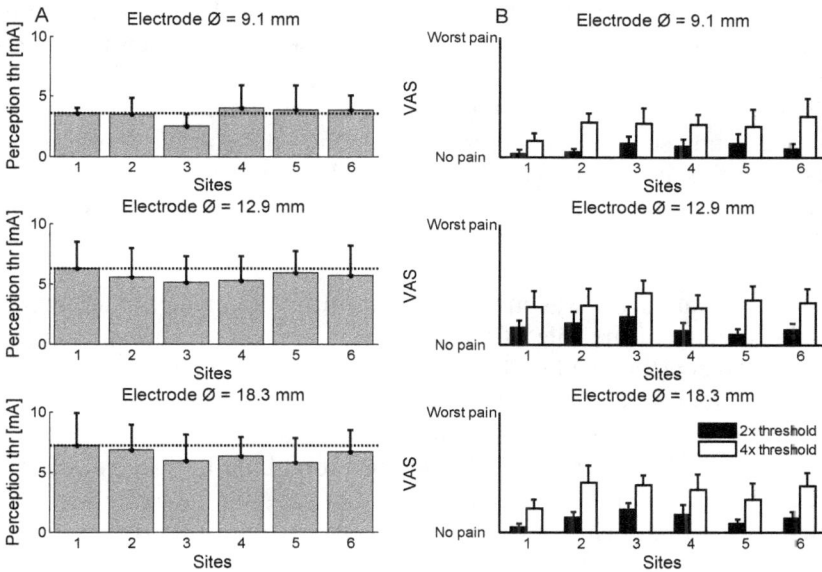

Figure 10. A) Perception threshold (mA) for stimulation using three electrode sizes (mean ± SD). The threshold increased significantly with electrode radius (RM ANOVA, p < 0.001). B) VAS scores for all stimulation sites and electrode sizes (mean ± SD). VAS scores did not vary across electrode sizes or stimulation sites (log transformed, RM ANOVA, NS). VAS scores were significantly higher when stimulating at the higher intensity (4x threshold) (log transformed, RM ANOVA, *p* < 0.05).

In *study II* three different electrode sizes were tested and figure 9 show that smaller electrodes will create a higher degree of $A\delta$ fiber activation, which is in agreement with previous studies (Kuhn et al. 2010; Morch et al. 2011). Furthermore, higher stimulus intensity also caused a higher degree of $A\delta$

fiber activation. This is not surprising since the Aδ fibers primarily functions as a nociceptor and it is activated by noxious stimulus.

4.3.2 Volume conductor modeling of electrical stimulation at the foot (study II & III)

Previous studies focusing on the NWR have hypothesized that part of the very inhomogeneous reflex response across the sole of the foot is due to differences in skin thickness (Andersen et al. 2004). Intuitively this makes very good sense, as it is clear that skin at the heel is extremely thick compared to the arch of the foot. This thicker skin would then insulate the deeper cutaneous receptors from the high energy stimulus. This might also explain why stimulations at the heel sometimes are perceived as less localized and sometimes spreading around the heel. Therefore, to investigate this in detail a number of models were developed to simulate the electrical stimulation in the sole of the foot. But before developing these models, the thicknesses of the various tissues types were determined (figure 11).

The volume conductor was modeled using the finite element method. The model geometry of the sole of the foot was based on the measurements of the tissue layers (figure 11). The geometry of the dorsum and lateral/medial sides of the foot was based on previous data from the literature (Kuhn et al. 2009; Morch et al. 2011). One surprising finding was that the current appears to mainly flow through the dermis around the foot to the reference electrode (figure 12), meaning that the more resistive fat layer acts as an electric isolator. The model was validated using experimental measurements of the impedances between the stimulation and reference electrodes. Generally, the model suggested higher impedances than found experimentally. This is very likely to be caused by two factors. First, the electrodes used in the experiments were 'wet' meaning they had a small layer of highly conductive gel which undoubtedly will diffuse into the skin and hence lower the impedance. This in-diffusion of the gel could not easily be simulated in the model. Secondly, the skin was abraded slightly to reduce the impedance prior to electrode placement – which is normal NWR practice (Andersen et al. 1999; Neziri et al. 2009) and necessary to realistically investigate the neural activation. Reducing the impedance of stratum corneum in the model led to better agreement between model and experiments. Thus, the model was considered validated.

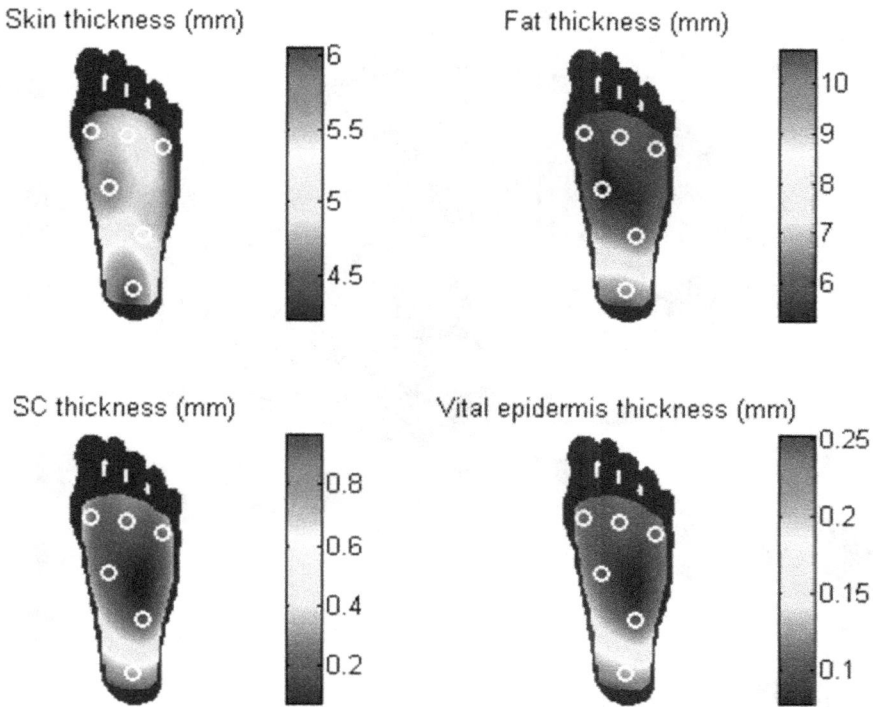

Figure 11. Interpolation maps of the measured thickness of different tissue types. The heel generally has higher average tissue thickness compared to the rest of the sole of the foot. The thickness of the dermis was deducted from the thickness of the entire skin, subtracted the thickness of the SC and vital epidermis. The muscles thickness was also measured, but is not depicted. Note that only the sites (white circles) express the exact measured thickness of the tissue. The maps were developed using a spline interpolation algorithm between the six sites.

Besides investigating the volume conductor itself the model was also used to describe the extracellular potentials leading to neural activation.

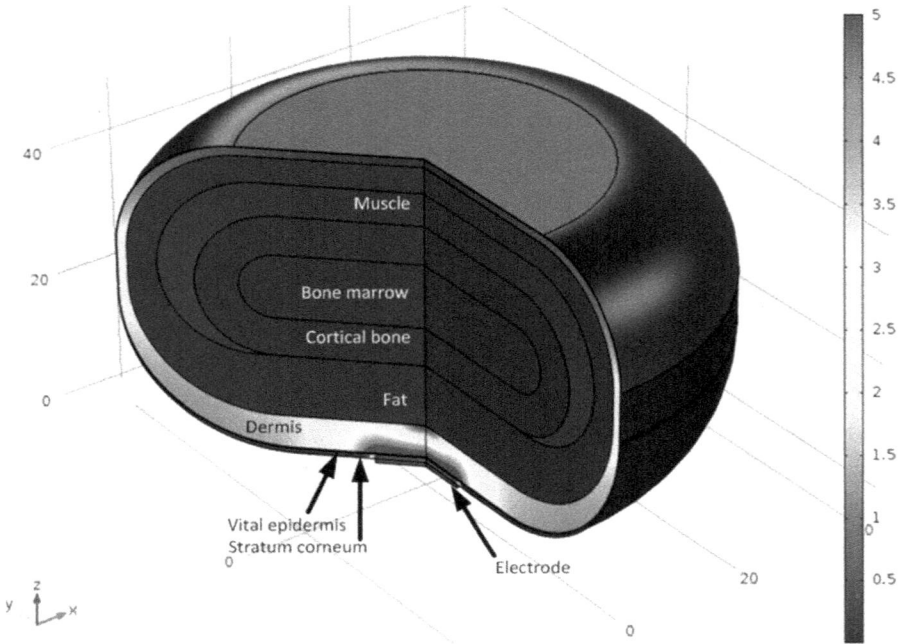

Figure 12. 3D current flow in the volume conductor model. The axisymmetric model was rotated and cut to show the 3D extent of the model and how the current flows through the tissue during a 1 mA stimulation. The color scale indicates the current density (A/m^2) and it was truncated at 5 A/m^2. The spatial grid is indicated in mm.

4.4 Models of the neural activation in the sole of the foot (study II & III)

Models of the activation of cutaneous nerves were used to investigate the experimentally found differences in neural activation. The activation function (AF) was calculated directly from the volume conductor model.

The AF showed that the difference in the volume conductor could be the cause for the difference seen across the sole of the foot (figure 13). However, this is at best a rough estimate. A more anatomically correct model of the nerve morphology was applied for further investigation. The applied model was an updated version of a previous model (Morch et al. 2011) inspired by the work of McNeal (McNeal 1976).

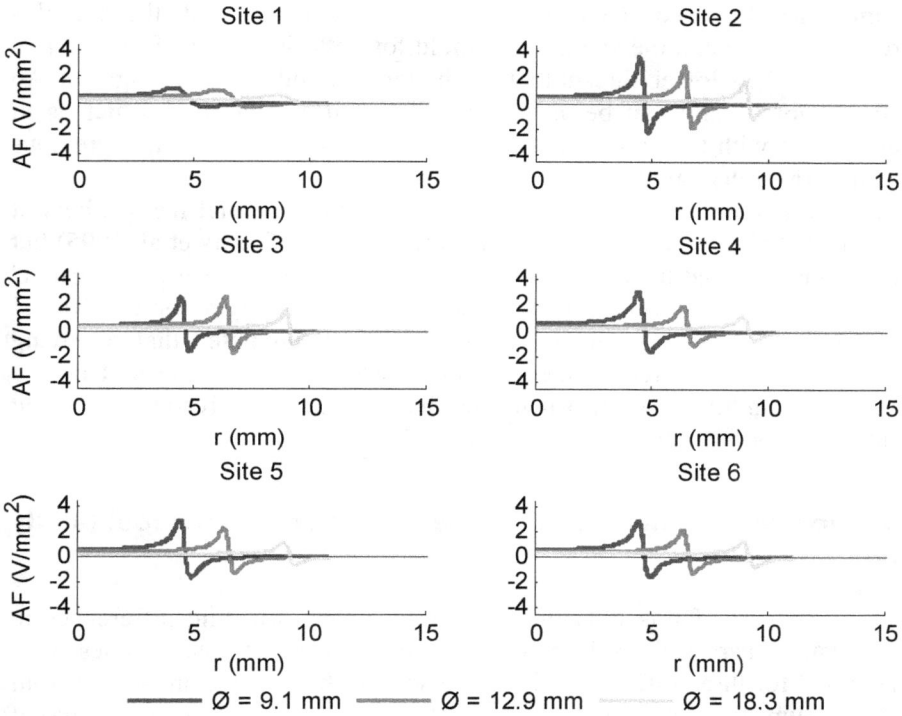

Figure 13. The calculated activation function (AF) along the dermo-epidermal ridge. The figure depicts the AF for the six sites and three electrode sizes used in *study II*. The AF was highest at the edges of the electrodes. Generally, the AF follows the same pattern for all modeled combinations. However, the absolute values at the heel (site 1) are considerably smaller than all other sites. Positive values indicate likely neural activation, negative indicate likely neural inhibition.

The cable model of the neural activation featured a realistic representation of the morphology of the cutaneous Aβ and Aδ fibers. Based on the combination of the volume conductor model and the cable model, the activation threshold for the fibers could be extracted. In contrast to the AF this model showed minor differences across the sole of the foot (figure 14). The stimulus-response function for both the Aβ and Aδ fibers were very similar across the tested sites, and for most cases fitted well with previous experimental values of perception and pain threshold (Andersen et al.

2004). Regarding the varying electrode sizes there was a clear and significant difference (ANOVA, p < 0.001) between both the stimulus response curve and the average threshold for both fiber types. Both $A\beta$ and $A\delta$ fibers had lower threshold for smaller electrodes, indicating that $A\delta$ fibers more easily can be activated with smaller electrodes, which is in agreement with the experimental findings in this project and also previous studies (Morch et al. 2011).

The nerve stainings found no evidence for intraepidermal nerve fibers at the heel. This is in contrast to previous findings (McCarthy et al. 1995) but could indicate that the previously found IENFs at the heel were primarily C fibers and *not* $A\delta$ fibers, which was the primary target for the $Na_v1.7$ stainings in this study. Interestingly, the model predicted that removing these IENFs would reduce the threshold, instead of increasing it. This is a bit counterintuitive because it means that the site of activation is located further away from the stimulation electrode.

4.5 Nociceptive innervation of the human sole of the foot (study III)

The final part of this PhD thesis focused on investigating differences in innervation across the sole of the foot. Post mortem tissue samples were obtained for three different sites in the sole of the foot (figure 4) and from the dorsum. Both staining techniques (Sihler and $Na_v 1.7$) were capable of identifying several nerves in the cutaneous tissue from the sole of the foot. Only the sodium channel antibody ($Na_v1.7$) was used to stain nerves from the dorsum. The results showed no significant differences in the innervation density across the sole of the foot (see figure 4 from *study III*). For the $Na_v1.7$ stainings, the densities in dorsum were significantly higher than those from the heel (ANOVA, p < 0.05) and arch (ANOVA, p < 0.01). This fits well with previous studies which reported that the innervation density in the sole is lower than other areas of the body (McCarthy et al. 1995).

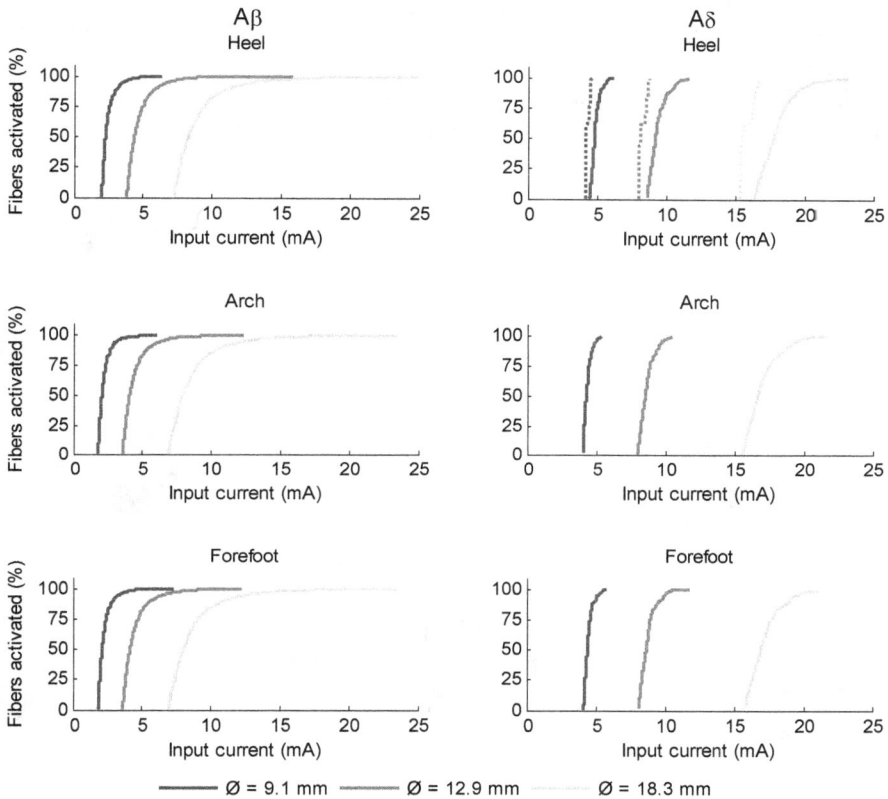

Figure 14. Stimulus – responses curves for the neural model. Generally the Aδ fibers had higher threshold than the Aβ fibers. By decreasing the electrode sizes (color codings) the activation threshold was reduced, which is in good agreement with the experiments conducted in this PhD project. The dotted lines for the Aδ fibers at the heel indicate models without IENFs. The removal of the IENFs would reduce the activation threshold comparing to the model including the IENFs (full lines).

The cable model of the neural activation was adjusted according to these findings. However, the combination of the anatomical study and the models did not conclusively reveal the background for the differences in perception and reflex excitability seen across the sole of the foot. Hence, the differences in reflex excitability are not purely caused by the investigated peripheral mechanisms. A central component is an alternative which makes sense since sudden reflexes, e.g. during gait, could perturb balance and upright posture and could therefore cause a person to fall thus risking even greater injuries than what was been exposed at the heel. Therefore, the nociceptive input from especially the heel, may be filtered somewhat to ensure stable weight bearing and maintain intended movements.

Conclusions

This PhD thesis has investigated methods to improve the strategy for recording and eliciting the human NWR. *Study I* has shown how it is possible to reduce EMG crosstalk during reflex recordings and thus potentially improve the specificity of the reflex recording. *Study II* documented and investigated how stimulation in the sole of the foot results in different levels of neural activation as an explanation for variation in reflex excitability. *Study III* investigated peripheral mechanisms as the background for the differences found in *study II*, but did not discover any evidence indicating peripheral explanations for the varying reflex excitability. Both *study II* and *III* found that several parameters affect the neural activation, especially the electrode size; however, neither *study II* or *III* could conclusively suggest methods for improved stimulation parameters/paradigm.

5.1 Implications

The major implication from *study I* was the recommendation of using DD sEMG recordings instead of SD. One drawback of DD recordings is that the signal-to-noise ratio might decrease; however, this did not seem to affect the single-channel recordings. Therefore, the combination of DD recordings and a similar setup as the single channel recordings appeared to be a way of improving the method for recording the NWR. The main contribution from *study II* was the confirmation of what appeared to be differences in neural activation across the sole of the foot following electrical stimulation. *Study II* also developed a volume conductor model, based on the finite element method, which gave insight in the current flow between the cathode and anode electrodes. *Study II* showed indications of peripheral mechanisms as the background for the differences in reflex

39

excitability; however, this was more thoroughly investigated in *study III*. *Study III* was a direct continuation of *study II* and found that the differences in perception observed in *study II* could not be explained by purely peripheral mechanisms like innervation differences or differences in tissue thickness across the sole. The discovery of what appeared to be differences in Aδ fiber activation might be reduced by the use of smaller electrodes, since *study II* and *III* showed this might result in a higher degree of Aδ activation. Therefore, smaller electrodes may be capable of lowering the NWR threshold but at the same time, a degree of spatial summation (concurrent activation of Aδ fibers from a confined area) is needed for evoking the reflex, limiting the area reduction of the electrode. However, smaller electrodes will also be associated with increased impedance which may result in a compliance problem for the constant current stimulators. This could in theory be solved by developing new stimulators with higher voltage compliance than the ones used in this PhD thesis. However, this is not a particularly safe approach. Therefore, it is recommended to use as small electrodes as possible within the compliance level of available stimulators.

The lack of evidence for the investigated peripheral mechanisms as the background for the different perception and reflex excitability could indicate a possible central component gating the afferent input from the sole of the foot. If present, such a central component would appear to primarily modulate reflexes in the triceps surae group by stimulation in the heel. The suggestion of a central component fits well with the fact that reflexes at the heel may likely be conveyed through more synapses (Andersen et al. 1999). The sole of the foot and especially the heel has to withstand significant strain during gait and upright posture and 'unwanted' reflexes might disturb the balance, resulting in falls and potentially injuries. If there exists a central component modulating the NWRs elicited from the heel, it may be advantageous to study the NWR using primarily other areas of the sole of the foot to elicit reflexes in muscles like TA or peroneus longus as already done in some NWR studies (Bjerre et al. 2011).

Future work

The findings in *study I* should be applied experimentally to remap the RRFs to test whether the use of DD can in fact reduce the variability and increase the validity of the RRF. *Study II* and *III* did not reveal any direct way of improving the methodology behind NWR elicitation. However, the studies did improve the knowledge of the underlying mechanisms for reflex elicitation. Future research should be based on these findings, for example the investigation of a possible central component. Besides the use of graded electrode sizes it may also be worth to investigate the general configuration, e.g. the use of a large common anode at the dorsum. No doubt the electrodes located at the heel are located the furthest away from the anode compared to the rest of the stimulating electrodes in the sole. This may have a small effect on the neural activation and was not simulated in the developed models. In order to test this, other electrode configurations could be used, e.g. a concentric electrode where the anode/stimulating electrode is placed in the center and the cathode/reference is placed surrounding the center. This would give a more localized current spread, only present in the sole of the foot.

To sum up, this PhD thesis has found ways of potentially improving the method for recording the NWR and hence the validity of the RRF assessments. Furthermore, it has shed light on the mechanisms underlying the elicitation of the NWR from different sites in the sole of the foot. However, some of the findings will require future research to understand and improve our understanding of the reflex neurophysiology.

References

Andersen, O. K. 2007, "Studies of the organization of the human nociceptive withdrawal reflex. Focus on sensory convergence and stimulation site dependency", *Acta Physiol (Oxf).*, vol. 189, no. 654, pp. 1-35.

Andersen, O. K., Finnerup, N. B., Spaich, E. G., Jensen, T. S., & Arendt-Nielsen, L. 2004, "Expansion of nociceptive withdrawal reflex receptive fields in spinal cord injured humans", *Clin.Neurophysiol.*, vol. 115, no. 12, pp. 2798-2810.

Andersen, O. K., Sonnenborg, F. A., & Arendt-Nielsen, L. 1999, "Modular organization of human leg withdrawal reflexes elicited by electrical stimulation of the foot sole", *Muscle Nerve.*, vol. 22, no. 11, pp. 1520-1530.

Andersen, O. K., Sonnenborg, F. A., & Arendt-Nielsen, L. 2001, "Reflex receptive fields for human withdrawal reflexes elicited by non-painful and painful electrical stimulation of the foot sole", *Clin.Neurophysiol.*, vol. 112, no. 4, pp. 641-649.

Andersen, O. K., Sonnenborg, F. A., Matjacic, Z., & Arendt-Nielsen, L. 2003, "Foot-sole reflex receptive fields for human withdrawal reflexes in symmetrical standing position", *Exp.Brain Res.*, vol. 152, no. 4, pp. 434-443.

Andersen, O. K., Spaich, E. G., Madeleine, P., & Arendt-Nielsen, L. 2005, "Gradual enlargement of human withdrawal reflex receptive fields following repetitive painful stimulation", *Brain Res.*, vol. 1042, no. 2, pp. 194-204.

Bjerre, L., Andersen, A. T., Hagelskjaer, M. T., Ge, N., Morch, C. D., & Andersen, O. K. 2011, "Dynamic tuning of human withdrawal reflex receptive fields during cognitive attention and distraction tasks", *Eur.J.Pain*, vol. 15, no. 8, pp. 816-821.

Black, J. A., Frezel, N., Dib-Hajj, S. D., & Waxman, S. G. 2012, "Expression of Nav1.7 in DRG neurons extends from peripheral terminals in the skin to central preterminal branches and terminals in the dorsal horn", *Mol.Pain*, vol. 8, p. 82.

Black, J. A., Renganathan, M., & Waxman, S. G. 2002, "Sodium channel Na(v)1.6 is expressed along nonmyelinated axons and it contributes to conduction", *Brain Res.Mol.Brain Res.*, vol. 105, no. 1-2, pp. 19-28.

Blyth, F. M., March, L. M., Brnabic, A. J., Jorm, L. R., Williamson, M., & Cousins, M. J. 2001, "Chronic pain in Australia: a prevalence study", *Pain.*, vol. 89, no. 2-3, pp. 127-134.

Catterall, W. A., Goldin, A. L., & Waxman, S. G. 2005, "International Union of Pharmacology. XLVII. Nomenclature and structure-function relationships of voltage-gated sodium channels", *Pharmacol.Rev.*, vol. 57, no. 4, pp. 397-409.

De Luca, C. J. & Merletti, R. 1988, "Surface myoelectric signal cross-talk among muscles of the leg", *Electroencephalogr.Clin.Neurophysiol.*, vol. 69, no. 6, pp. 568-575.

Dib-Hajj, S. D., Black, J. A., & Waxman, S. G. 2009, "Voltage-gated sodium channels: therapeutic targets for pain", *Pain Med.*, vol. 10, no. 7, pp. 1260-1269.

Drewes, A. M., Helweg-Larsen, S., Petersen, P., Brennum, J., Andreasen, A., Poulsen, L. H., & Jensen, T. S. 1993, "McGill Pain Questionnaire translated into Danish: experimental and clinical findings", *Clin.J.Pain.*, vol. 9, no. 2, pp. 80-87.

Ebenezer, G. J., Hauer, P., Gibbons, C., McArthur, J. C., & Polydefkis, M. 2007, "Assessment of epidermal nerve fibers: a new diagnostic and predictive tool for peripheral neuropathies", *J.Neuropathol.Exp.Neurol.*, vol. 66, no. 12, pp. 1059-1073.

Eriksen, J. & Sjogren, P. 2006, "[Epidemiological factors relating to long-term/chronic non-cancer pain in Denmark]", *Ugeskr.Laeger.*, vol. 168, no. 20, pp. 1947-1950.

Farina, D. 2006, "Interpretation of the surface electromyogram in dynamic contractions", *Exerc.Sport Sci.Rev.*, vol. 34, no. 3, pp. 121-127.

Farina, D., Merletti, R., & Enoka, R. M. 2004a, "The extraction of neural strategies from the surface EMG", *J.Appl.Physiol.*, vol. 96, no. 4, pp. 1486-1495.

Farina, D., Merletti, R., Indino, B., & Graven-Nielsen, T. 2004b, "Surface EMG crosstalk evaluated from experimental recordings and simulated signals. Reflections on crosstalk interpretation, quantification and reduction", *Methods Inf.Med.*, vol. 43, no. 1, pp. 30-35.

Farina, D., Merletti, R., Indino, B., Nazzaro, M., & Pozzo, M. 2002, "Surface EMG crosstalk between knee extensor muscles: experimental and model results", *Muscle Nerve.*, vol. 26, no. 5, pp. 681-695.

Floeter, M. K., Gerloff, C., Kouri, J., & Hallett, M. 1998, "Cutaneous withdrawal reflexes of the upper extremity", *Muscle Nerve*, vol. 21, no. 5, pp. 591-598.

Frahm, K. S., Andersen, O. K., Arendt-Nielsen, L., & Morch, C. D. 2010, "Spatial temperature distribution in human hairy and glabrous skin after infrared CO_2 laser radiation", *Biomed.Eng Online.*, vol. 9, p. 69.

Frahm, K. S., Jensen, M. B., Farina, D., & Andersen, O. K. 2012, "Surface EMG crosstalk during phasic involuntary muscle activation in the nociceptive withdrawal reflex", *Muscle Nerve.*, vol. 46, no. 2, pp. 228-236.

France, C. R., Rhudy, J. L., & McGlone, S. 2009, "Using normalized EMG to define the nociceptive flexion reflex (NFR) threshold: further evaluation of standardized NFR scoring criteria", *Pain.*, vol. 145, no. 1-2, pp. 211-218.

Gabriel, S., Lau, R. W., & Gabriel, C. 1996, "The dielectric properties of biological tissues: II. Measurements in the frequency range 10 Hz to 20 GHz", *Phys.Med.Biol.*, vol. 41, no. 11, pp. 2251-2269.

Gracely, R. H. 1999, "Studies of pain in human subjects," in *Textbook of Pain*, P. D. Wall & R. Melzack, eds., pp. 385-408.

Grill, W. M. 1999, "Modeling the effects of electric fields on nerve fibers: influence of tissue electrical properties", *IEEE Trans.Biomed.Eng.*, vol. 46, no. 8, pp. 918-928.

Grimby, L. 1963, "Normal plantar response: integration of flexor and extensor reflex components", *J.Neurol.Neurosurg.Psychiatry.*, vol. 26:39-50., pp. 39-50.

Hagbarth, K. E. 1960, "Spinal withdrawal reflexes in the human lower limbs", *J.Neurol.Neurosurg.Psychiatry.*, vol. 23:222-7., pp. 222-227.

Hansen, N., Klein, T., Magerl, W., & Treede, R. D. 2007, "Psychophysical evidence for long-term potentiation of C-fiber and Adelta-fiber pathways in humans by analysis of pain descriptors", *J.Neurophysiol.*, vol. 97, no. 3, pp. 2559-2563.

Hernandez-Plata, E., Ortiz, C. S., Marquina-Castillo, B., Medina-Martinez, I., Alfaro, A., Berumen, J., Rivera, M., & Gomora, J. C.

2012, "Overexpression of NaV 1.6 channels is associated with the invasion capacity of human cervical cancer", *Int.J.Cancer.*, vol. 130, no. 9, pp. 2013-2023.

Herzog, R. I., Cummins, T. R., Ghassemi, F., Dib-Hajj, S. D., & Waxman, S. G. 2003, "Distinct repriming and closed-state inactivation kinetics of Nav1.6 and Nav1.7 sodium channels in mouse spinal sensory neurons", *J.Physiol.*, vol. 551, no. Pt 3, pp. 741-750.

Hilliges, M., Wang, L., & Johansson, O. 1995, "Ultrastructural evidence for nerve fibers within all vital layers of the human epidermis", *J.Invest Dermatol.*, vol. 104, no. 1, pp. 134-137.

Hodgkin, A. L. & Huxley, A. F. 1952, "A quantitative description of membrane current and its application to conduction and excitation in nerve", *J.Physiol.*, vol. 117, no. 4, pp. 500-544.

Hugon, M. 1973, "Exteroceptive Reflexes to Stimulation of the Sural Nerve in Normal Man," in *New Developments in Electromygraphy and Clinical Neurophysiology*, 3 edn, J. E. Desmedt, ed., pp. 713-729.

Kennedy, P. M. & Inglis, J. T. 2002, "Distribution and behaviour of glabrous cutaneous receptors in the human foot sole", *J.Physiol.*, vol. 538, no. Pt 3, pp. 995-1002.

Kennedy, W. R. & Wendelschafer-Crabb, G. 1993, "The innervation of human epidermis", *J.Neurol.Sci.*, vol. 115, no. 2, pp. 184-190.

Kuhn, A., Keller, T., Lawrence, M., & Morari, M. 2009, "A model for transcutaneous current stimulation: simulations and experiments", *Med.Biol.Eng Comput.*, vol. 47, no. 3, pp. 279-289.

Kuhn, A., Keller, T., Lawrence, M., & Morari, M. 2010, "The influence of electrode size on selectivity and comfort in transcutaneous electrical stimulation of the forearm", *IEEE Trans.Neural Syst.Rehabil.Eng.*, vol. 18, no. 3, pp. 255-262.

Latremoliere, A. & Woolf, C. J. 2009, "Central sensitization: a generator of pain hypersensitivity by central neural plasticity", *J.Pain.*, vol. 10, no. 9, pp. 895-926.

Le, B. D., Gozariu, M., & Cadden, S. W. 2001, "Animal models of nociception", *Pharmacol.Rev.*, vol. 53, no. 4, pp. 597-652.

Loeser, J. D. & Treede, R. D. 2008, "The Kyoto protocol of IASP Basic Pain Terminology", *Pain.*, vol. 137, no. 3, pp. 473-477.

Maiani, G. & Sanavio, E. 1985, "Semantics of pain in Italy: the Italian version of the McGill Pain Questionnaire", *Pain.*, vol. 22, no. 4, pp. 399-405.

Manresa, J. A., Jensen, M. B., & Andersen, O. K. 2011, "Introducing the reflex probability maps in the quantification of nociceptive withdrawal reflex receptive fields in humans", *J.Electromyogr.Kinesiol.*, vol. 21, no. 1, pp. 67-76.

McCarthy, B. G., Hsieh, S. T., Stocks, A., Hauer, P., Macko, C., Cornblath, D. R., Griffin, J. W., & McArthur, J. C. 1995, "Cutaneous innervation in sensory neuropathies: evaluation by skin biopsy", *Neurology.*, vol. 45, no. 10, pp. 1848-1855.

McIntyre, C. C., Richardson, A. G., & Grill, W. M. 2002, "Modeling the excitability of mammalian nerve fibers: influence of afterpotentials on the recovery cycle", *J.Neurophysiol.*, vol. 87, no. 2, pp. 995-1006.

McNeal, D. R. 1976, "Analysis of a model for excitation of myelinated nerve", *IEEE Trans.Biomed.Eng.*, vol. 23, no. 4, pp. 329-337.

Melzack, R. 1975, "The McGill Pain Questionnaire: major properties and scoring methods", *Pain.*, vol. 1, no. 3, pp. 277-299.

Melzack, R. 1987, "The short-form McGill Pain Questionnaire", *Pain.*, vol. 30, no. 2, pp. 191-197.

Mesin, L., Smith, S., Hugo, S., Viljoen, S., & Hanekom, T. 2009, "Effect of spatial filtering on crosstalk reduction in surface EMG recordings", *Med.Eng Phys.*, vol. 31, no. 3, pp. 374-383.

Morch, C. D., Andersen, O. K., Graven-Nielsen, T., & Arendt-Nielsen, L. 2007, "Nociceptive withdrawal reflexes evoked by uniform-temperature laser heat stimulation of large skin areas in humans", *J.Neurosci.Methods.*, vol. 160, no. 1, pp. 85-92.

Morch, C. D., Hennings, K., & Andersen, O. K. 2011, "Estimating nerve excitation thresholds to cutaneous electrical stimulation by finite element modeling combined with a stochastic branching nerve fiber model", *Med.Biol.Eng Comput.*, vol. 49, pp. 385-395.

Neziri, A. Y., Andersen, O. K., Petersen-Felix, S., Radanov, B., Dickenson, A. H., Scaramozzino, P., Arendt-Nielsen, L., & Curatolo, M. 2010, "The nociceptive withdrawal reflex: normative values of thresholds and reflex receptive fields", *Eur.J.Pain.*, vol. 14, no. 2, pp. 134-141.

Neziri, A. Y., Curatolo, M., Bergadano, A., Petersen-Felix, S., Dickenson, A. H., Arendt-Nielsen, L., & Andersen, O. K. 2009, "New method for quantification and statistical analysis of nociceptive reflex receptive fields in humans", *J.Neurosci.Methods.*, vol. 178, no. 1, pp. 24-30.

Panizza, M., Nilsson, J., Roth, B. J., Grill, S. E., Demirci, M., & Hallett, M. 1998, "Differences between the time constant of sensory and motor peripheral nerve fibers: further studies and considerations", *Muscle Nerve.*, vol. 21, no. 1, pp. 48-54.

Perrotta, A., Serpino, C., Cormio, C., Serrao, M., Sandrini, G., Pierelli, F., & de, T. M. 2012, "Abnormal spinal cord pain processing in Huntington's disease. The role of the diffuse noxious inhibitory control", *Clin.Neurophysiol.*, vol. 123, no. 8, pp. 1624-1630.

Persson, A. K., Black, J. A., Gasser, A., Cheng, X., Fischer, T. Z., & Waxman, S. G. 2010, "Sodium-calcium exchanger and multiple sodium channel isoforms in intra-epidermal nerve terminals", *Mol.Pain.*, vol. 6:84., p. 84.

Rattay, F. 1986, "Analysis of models for external stimulation of axons", *IEEE Trans.Biomed.Eng.*, vol. 33, no. 10, pp. 974-977.

Reilly, D. M., Ferdinando, D., Johnston, C., Shaw, C., Buchanan, K. D., & Green, M. R. 1997, "The epidermal nerve fibre network: characterization of nerve fibres in human skin by confocal microscopy and assessment of racial variations", *Br.J.Dermatol.*, vol. 137, no. 2, pp. 163-170.

Reilly, J. P., Freeman, V. T., & Larkin, W. D. 1985, "Sensory effects of transient electrical stimulation--evaluation with a neuroelectric model", *IEEE Trans.Biomed.Eng.*, vol. 32, no. 12, pp. 1001-1011.

Rhudy, J. L. & France, C. R. 2007, "Defining the nociceptive flexion reflex (NFR) threshold in human participants: a comparison of different scoring criteria", *Pain.*, vol. 128, no. 3, pp. 244-253.

Sandrini, G., Serrao, M., Rossi, P., Romaniello, A., Cruccu, G., & Willer, J. C. 2005, "The lower limb flexion reflex in humans", *Prog.Neurobiol.*, vol. 77, no. 6, pp. 353-395.

Schouenborg, J. & Kalliomaki, J. 1990, "Functional organization of the nociceptive withdrawal reflexes. I. Activation of hindlimb muscles in the rat", *Exp.Brain Res.*, vol. 83, no. 1, pp. 67-78.

Schouenborg, J. & Weng, H. R. 1994, "Sensorimotor transformation in a spinal motor system", *Exp.Brain Res.*, vol. 100, no. 1, pp. 170-174.

Schouenborg, J., Weng, H. R., Kalliomaki, J., & Holmberg, H. 1995, "A survey of spinal dorsal horn neurones encoding the spatial organization of withdrawal reflexes in the rat", *Exp.Brain Res.*, vol. 106, no. 1, pp. 19-27.

Sherrington, C. S. 1910, "Flexion-reflex of the limb, crossed extension-reflex, and reflex stepping and standing", *J.Physiol.*, vol. 40, no. 1-2, pp. 28-121.

Skljarevski, V. & Ramadan, N. M. 2002, "The nociceptive flexion reflex in humans -- review article", *Pain.*, vol. 96, no. 1-2, pp. 3-8.

Sonnenborg, F. A., Andersen, O. K., & Arendt-Nielsen, L. 2000, "Modular organization of excitatory and inhibitory reflex receptive fields elicited by electrical stimulation of the foot sole in man", *Clin.Neurophysiol.*, vol. 111, no. 12, pp. 2160-2169.

Sonnenborg, F. A., Andersen, O. K., Arendt-Nielsen, L., & Treede, R. D. 2001, "Withdrawal reflex organisation to electrical stimulation of the dorsal foot in humans", *Exp.Brain Res.*, vol. 136, no. 3, pp. 303-312.

Tavernier, A., Dierickx, M., & Hinsenkamp, M. 1993, "Tensors of dielectric permittivity and conductivity of in vitro human derms and epiderms.", *Bioelectroch.Bioener.*, vol. 30, pp. 65-72.

Terry, E. L., France, C. R., Bartley, E. J., Delventura, J. L., Kerr, K. L., Vincent, A. L., & Rhudy, J. L. 2011, "Standardizing procedures to study sensitization of human spinal nociceptive processes: comparing parameters for temporal summation of the nociceptive flexion reflex (TS-NFR)", *Int.J.Psychophysiol.*, vol. 81, no. 3, pp. 263-274.

Tørring, J., Pedersen, E., & Klemar, B. 1981, "Standardisation of the electrical elicitation of the human flexor reflex", *J.Neurol.Neurosurg.Psychiatry.*, vol. 44, no. 2, pp. 129-132.

Tu, H., Zhang, L., Tran, T. P., Muelleman, R. L., & Li, Y. L. 2010, "Reduced expression and activation of voltage-gated sodium channels contributes to blunted baroreflex sensitivity in heart failure rats", *J.Neurosci.Res.*, vol. 88, no. 15, pp. 3337-3349.

van Vugt, J. P. & van Dijk, J. G. 2001, "A convenient method to reduce crosstalk in surface EMG. Cobb Award-winning article, 2001", *Clin.Neurophysiol.*, vol. 112, no. 4, pp. 583-592.

Woolf, C. J. 1983, "Evidence for a central component of post-injury pain hypersensitivity", *Nature.*, vol. 306, no. 5944, pp. 686-688.

Yamamoto, T. & Yamamoto, Y. 1976, "Electrical properties of the epidermal stratum corneum", *Med.Biol.Eng.*, vol. 14, no. 2, pp. 151-158.

About the author

Ken Steffen Frahm was born in Hammel, Denmark June 19th 1983. He graduated as a biomedical engineer (M.Sc. BME) in June 2009 after having followed the elite scholar program at Aalborg University, Denmark. From September 2009 to march 2013 he was enrolled as a PhD student at the Center for Sensory-Motor Interaction at Aalborg University. His primary research interests are pain and neurophysiological research especially within electrophysiology and physiological modeling.

www.ingramcontent.com/pod-product-compliance
Lightning Source LLC
Chambersburg PA
CBHW061840220326
41599CB00027B/5352